the unwinding of the miracle

A memoir of life, death, and everything that comes after

JULIE YIP-WILLIAMS

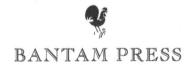

BANTAM PRESS

TRANSWORLD PUBLISHERS
61–63 Uxbridge Road, London W5 5SA
www.penguin.co.uk

Transworld is part of the Penguin Random House group of companies
whose addresses can be found at global.penguinrandomhouse.com

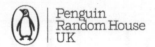

First published in Great Britain in 2019 by Bantam Press
an imprint of Transworld Publishers

Portions of this work were originally published, sometimes in different
form, on the author's blog, julieyipwilliams.wordpress.com

Every effort has been made to obtain the necessary permissions with
reference to copyright material, both illustrative and quoted. We apologize
for any omissions in this respect and will be pleased to make the
appropriate acknowledgements in any future edition.

A CIP catalogue record for this book
is available from the British Library.

ISBN 9781787630406

Typeset in 11.16/14.73 pt Dante MT Std by Jouve (UK), Milton Keynes
Printed and bound in Great Britain by Clays Ltd. Elcograf S.p.A.

Penguin Random House is committed to a sustainable future
for our business, our readers and our planet. This book is made
from Forest Stewardship Council® certified paper.

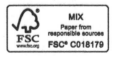

1 3 5 7 9 10 8 6 4 2

This book is dedicated to Josh, Mia, and Isabelle—
the loves of my life

to Lyna, Nancy, and Caroline—
my beloved sisterhood

to my parents, 葉世福 and 林桂英,
who did their best for me

and to my brother Mau,
who walked me safely down the street

the
unwinding
of the
miracle

www.penguin.co.uk

Contents

Prologue

Hello, welcome.

My name is Julie Yip-Williams. I am grateful and deeply honored that you are here. This story begins at the ending. Which means that if you are here, then I am not. But it's okay.

My life was good and my life was complete. It came to so much more than I ever thought possible, or than my very humble beginnings would have given me the right to expect. I was a wife, a mother, a daughter, a sister, a friend, an immigrant, a cancer patient, a lawyer, and now a writer. I tried to live always with good intentions and a good heart, although I am sure I have hurt people along the way. I tried my best to live a full, rewarding life, to deal with the inevitable trials with grace, and to emerge with my sense of humor and love for life intact. That's all. Even though I am dying in my early forties, and leaving my precious children behind, I am happy.

My life was not easy. That I survived infancy was something of a miracle, that I made it to America, also a miracle. Being born poor and blind in Vietnam on the losing side of a bloody civil war should have defined my life and sealed my fate. Those things marked me, but they did not stop me. Dying has taught me a great deal about living—about facing hard truths consciously, about embracing the suffering as well as the joy. Wrapping my arms around the hard parts was perhaps the great liberating experience of my life.

Directly or indirectly, we all experience the hard parts. The events that we hear about on the news or from friends, those tragedies ending in death that happen to other people in other places, which make us sad but also relieved and grateful as we think, There but for the grace of God . . . —destructive hurricanes and earthquakes, violent shootings and explosions, car accidents, and of course, insidious illnesses. These things shake us to the core because they remind us of our mortality, of how impotent we truly are in the face of unseen forces that would cause the earth to tremble or cells to mutate and send a body into full rebellion against itself.

I set out here to write about my experience of that, both the life lived and the trials endured—neither comprehensively, you understand, but enough to fully show you the distance I traveled and the world in which I made my life. And what began as a chronicle of an early and imminent death became—if I may be very presumptuous—something far more meaningful: an exhortation to you, the living.

Live while you're living, friends.

From the beginning of the miracle, to the unwinding of the miracle.

JULIE YIP-WILLIAMS
February 2018

the
unwinding
of the
miracle

1

Death, Part One

March 1976, Tam Ky, South Vietnam

When I was two months old, my parents, on orders from my paternal grandmother, took me to an herbalist in Da Nang and offered the old man gold bars to give me a concoction that would make me sleep forever. Because I was born blind, to my Chinese grandmother, I was broken. I would be a burden and an embarrassment to the family. Unmarriageable. Besides, my grandmother reasoned, she was showing me mercy—I would be spared a miserable existence.

That morning, my mother dressed me in old baby clothes soiled with brownish-yellow stains from my sister's or brother's shit that she had not been able to wash away, even after countless scrubbings. My grandmother had ordered my mother to put me in these clothes and now stood in the doorway to my parents' bedroom, watching my mother dress me. "It would be a waste for her to wear anything else," she said when my mother was finished, as if to confirm the rightness of her instruction.

These were the clothes in which I was to die. In desperate times such as those, there was no point in throwing away a perfectly good baby outfit on an infant that was soon to become a corpse.

Our family drama played out in the red-hot center of the Cold War. South Vietnam had been "liberated" by the North eleven months earlier, and a geopolitical domino came crashing into the lives of the Yips.

By 1972, the war had turned decidedly against the South, and my father was terrified of losing what few possessions he had risking his life for a country for which he, as an ethnic Chinese man, felt little to no nationalistic pride. In his four years of military service, my father never talked to anyone in his family during his brief home leaves about what horrible things he had seen or done. His mother's attempts to spare him the ugliness of war by using bribery to get him a position as a driver for an army captain had not been as successful as they had all hoped. He found himself driving into enemy territory, uncertain where the snipers and land mines lurked, and sleeping in the jungle at night, afraid of the stealthy Vietcong slitting his throat while he slept on the jungle floor, and then jerking into motion by explosions that ripped open the silence of a tenuous calm. In the end, the constant fear of death—or, worse yet, of losing a limb, as had happened to some of his friends—overwhelmed whatever notions he had of honor and his fears of being labeled a coward. One day, he walked away from camp on the pretext of retrieving supplies from his jeep and didn't look back. For a week, he walked and hitchhiked his way to Saigon, the capital of South Vietnam, where he hid in Cholon, an old district inhabited by at least a million ethnic Chinese. Cholon was a place with such bustling activity and such a large population of those not loyal to the war effort that he could hide while still being able to move freely about the community.

My grandmother, to whom my father managed to get word of his whereabouts, trusted no man's ability to remain faithful, including her son's, and suggested to my mother that she join my father in Saigon. And so my mother, with my two-year-old sister, Lyna, in one arm and my infant brother, Mau, in the other, went to Saigon, and there they lived in limbo with my father until the end of the war, waiting until it was safe for him to return to Tam Ky without the fear of being imprisoned or, even worse, forced to continue military service in a rapidly deteriorating situation. It was not the time to have another child.

When Saigon fell on April 30, 1975, my parents rejoiced with the rest of Saigon, not because they believed in the new Communist regime but because the war was finally coming to an end. As Saigon changed hands, they celebrated by joining the feverish mobs ransacking abandoned stores and warehouses, taking tanks of gas and sacks of rice and whatever else their hands could carry away. They celebrated by welcoming the news of my pending arrival into this world, and after Saigon fell, they finally went home to Tam Ky, where I came into the world on an unremarkable January evening eight months later. I weighed a little more than three kilograms (between six and seven pounds), big by Vietnamese standards, but not so big that my mother and I were at the risk of dying during childbirth. Hospitals were filthy, and cesareans were not an option in those days; no one knew how to perform them, except maybe in Saigon. My father named me 莉菁, which is pronounced "Lijing" in Mandarin Chinese and "Lising" in Hainanese Chinese, and translated literally means "Quintessence of Jasmine." My name was intended to convey a sense of vibrancy, vitality, and beauty. My mother, who had waited so long for a new baby, was thrilled. And so was my grandmother—at first, anyhow. Two months later, wrapped in my brother and sister's old baby clothes, I was in my father's arms, on a bus, making the two-hour trip north to Da Nang on Highway 1, sentenced to death.

2

Life

July 14, 2017, Brooklyn, New York

Dear Mia and Isabelle,

I have solved all the logistical problems resulting from my death that I can think of—I am hiring a very reasonably priced cook for you and Daddy; I have left a list of instructions about who your dentist is and when your school tuition needs to be paid and when to renew the violin rental contract and the identity of the piano tuner. In the coming days, I will make videos about all the ins and outs of the apartment, so that everyone knows where the air filters are and what kind of dog food Chipper eats. But I realized that these things are the low-hanging fruit, the easy-to-solve but relatively unimportant problems of the oh so mundane.

I realized that I would have failed you greatly as your mother if I did not try to ease your pain from my loss, if I didn't at least attempt to address what will likely be the greatest question of your young lives. You will forever be the kids whose mother died of cancer, have people looking at you with some combination of sympathy and pity (which you will no doubt resent, even if everyone means well). That fact of your mother dying will weave into the fabric of your lives like a glaring stain on an otherwise pristine tableau. You will ask as you look around at all the other people who still have their parents, Why did my mother have to get sick and die? It isn't fair, you will cry. And you will want so painfully for me to be there to hug you when your friend is mean to you, to look on as your ears are being pierced, to sit in the front row clapping loudly at your music recitals, to be that annoying parent insisting on another photo with the college graduate, to help you get dressed on your wedding day, to take your newborn babe from your arms so you can sleep. And every time you yearn for me, it will hurt all over again and you will wonder why.

I don't know if my words could ever ease your pain. But I would be remiss if I did not try.

My seventh-grade history teacher, Mrs. Olson, a batty eccentric but a phenomenal teacher, used to rebut our teenage protestations of "That's not fair!" (for example, when she sprang a pop quiz on us or when we played what was called the "Unfair" trivia game) with "Life is not fair. Get used to it!" Somehow, we grow up thinking that there should be fairness, that people should be treated fairly, that there should be equality of treatment as well as opportunity. That expectation must be derived from growing up in a rich country where the rule of law is so firmly entrenched. Even at the tender age of five, both of you were screaming about fairness as if it were some fundamental right (as in it wasn't fair that Belle got to go to see a movie when Mia did not). So perhaps those expectations of fairness and equity are also hardwired into the human psyche and our moral compass. I'm not sure.

What I do know for sure is that Mrs. Olson was right. Life is not fair. You would be foolish to expect fairness, at least when it comes to matters of life and death, matters outside the scope of the law, matters that cannot be engineered or manipulated by human effort, matters that are distinctly the domain of God or luck or fate or some other unknowable, incomprehensible force.

Although I did not grow up motherless, I suffered in a different way and understood at an age younger than yours that life is not fair. I looked at all the other kids who could drive and play tennis and who didn't have to use a magnifying glass to read, and it pained me in a way that maybe you can understand now. People looked at me with pity, too, which I loathed. I was denied opportunities, too; I was always the scorekeeper and never played in the games during PE. My mother didn't think it worthwhile to have me study Chinese after English school, as my siblings did, because she assumed I wouldn't be able to see the characters. (Of course, later on, I would study Chinese throughout college and study abroad and my Chinese would surpass my siblings'.) For a child, there is nothing worse than being different, in that negative, pitiful way. I was sad a lot. I cried in my lonely anger. Like you, I had my own loss, the loss of vision, which involved the loss of so much more. I grieved. I asked why. I hated the unfairness of it all.

My sweet babies, I do not have the answer to the question of why, at least not now and not in this life. But I do know that there is incredible value in pain and suffering, if you allow yourself to experience it, to cry, to feel sorrow and grief, to hurt. Walk through the fire and you will emerge on the other end, whole and stronger. I promise. You will ultimately find truth and beauty and wisdom and peace. You will understand that nothing lasts forever, not pain, or joy. You will understand that joy cannot exist without sadness. Relief cannot exist without pain. Compassion cannot exist without cruelty. Courage cannot exist without fear. Hope cannot exist without despair. Wisdom cannot exist without suffering. Gratitude cannot exist without deprivation. Paradoxes abound in this life. Living is an exercise in navigating within them.

I was deprived of sight. And yet, that single unfortunate physical condition changed me for the better. Instead of leaving me wallowing in self-pity, it made me more ambitious. It made me more resourceful. It made me smarter. It taught me to ask for help, to not be ashamed of my physical shortcoming. It forced me to be honest with myself and my limitations, and eventually to be honest with others. It taught me strength and resilience.

You will be deprived of a mother. As your mother, I wish I could protect you from the pain. But also as your mother, I want you to feel the pain, to live it, embrace it, and then learn from it. Be stronger people because of it, for you will know that you carry my strength within you. Be more compassionate people because of it; empathize with those who suffer in their own ways. Rejoice in life and all its beauty because of it; live with special zest and zeal for me. Be grateful in a way that only someone who lost her mother so early can, in your understanding of the precariousness and preciousness of life. This is my challenge to you, my sweet girls, to take an ugly tragedy and transform it into a source of beauty, love, strength, courage, and wisdom.

Many may disagree, but I have always believed, always, even when I was a precocious little girl crying alone in my bed, that our purpose in this life is to experience everything we possibly can, to understand as much of the human condition as we can squeeze into one lifetime, however long or short that may be. We are here to feel the complex range of emotions that come with being human. And from those experiences, our souls expand and grow and learn and change, and we understand a little more about what it really means to be human. I call it the evolution of the soul. Know that your mother lived an incredible life that was filled with more than her "fair" share of pain and suffering, first with her blindness and then with cancer. And I allowed that pain and suffering to define me, to change me, but for the better.

In the years since my diagnosis, I have known love and compassion that I never knew possible; I have witnessed and experienced for myself the deepest levels of human caring, which humbled me to my core and compelled me to be a better person. I have known a mortal fear that was crushing, and yet I overcame that fear and found courage. The lessons that blindness and then cancer have taught me are too many for me to recount here, but I hope, when you read what follows, you will understand how it is possible to be changed in a positive way by tragedy and you will learn the true value of suffering. The worth of a person's life lies not in the number of years lived; rather it rests on how well that person has absorbed the lessons of that life, how well that person has come to understand and distill the multiple, messy aspects of the human experience. While I would have chosen to stay with you for much longer had the choice been mine, if you can learn from my death, if you accepted my challenge to be better people because of my death, then that would bring my spirit inordinate joy and peace.

You will feel alone and lonely, and yet, understand that you are not alone. It is true that we walk this life alone, because we feel what we feel singularly and each of us makes our own choices. But it is possible to reach out and find those like you, and in so doing you will feel not so lonely. This is another one of life's paradoxes that you will learn to navigate. First and foremost, you have each other to lean on. You are sisters, and that gives you a bond of blood and common experiences that is like no other. Find solace in one another. Always forgive and love one another. Then there's Daddy. Then there are Titi and Uncle Mau and Aunt Nancy and Aunt Caroline and Aunt Sue and so many dear friends, all of whom knew and loved me so well—who think of you and pray for you and worry about you. All of these people's loving energy surrounds you so that you will not feel so alone.

And last, wherever I may go, a part of me will always be with you. My blood flows within you. You have inherited the best parts of me. Even though I won't physically be here, I will be watching over you.

Sometimes, when you practice your instruments, I close my eyes so I can hear better. And when I do, I am often overcome with this absolute knowing that whenever you play the violin or the piano, when you play it with passion and commitment, the music with its special power will beckon me and I will be there. I will be sitting right there, pushing you to do it again and again and again, to count, to adjust your elbow, to sit properly. And then I will hug you and tell you how you did a great job and how very proud I am of you. I promise. Even long after you have chosen to stop playing, I will still come to you in those extraordinary and ordinary moments in life when you live with a complete passion and commitment. It might be while you're standing atop a mountain, marveling at exceptional beauty and filled with pride in your ability to reach the summit, or when you hold your baby in your arms for the first time or when you are crying because someone or something has broken your tender heart or maybe when you're miserably pulling an all-nighter for school or work. Know that your mother once felt as you feel and that I am there hugging you and urging you on. I promise.

I have often dreamed that when I die, I will finally know what it would be like to see the world without visual impairment, to see far into the distance, to see the minute details of a bird, to drive a car. Oh, how I long to have perfect vision, even after all these years without. I long for death to make me whole, to give me what was denied me in this life. I believe this dream will come true. Similarly, when your time comes, I will be there waiting for you, so that you, too, will be given what was lost to you. I promise. But in the meantime, live, my darling babies. Live a life worth living. Live thoroughly and completely, thoughtfully, gratefully, courageously, and wisely. Live!

I love you both forever and ever, to infinity, through space and time. Never ever forget that.

Mommy

Summer
and Fall
2013

3

The Odds

It was meant to be a family wedding. Midsummer 2013, everybody gathered in Los Angeles to celebrate my gorgeous young cousin's happiest day. I didn't make it. Josh and I had flown from New York with Mia and Belle, intending to stay about a week. For a month or so before that I had been having stomach discomfort—amorphous, other than that it just didn't feel normal. Nausea, cramping, and constipation had sent me to a gastroenterologist, but nothing appeared to be seriously amiss. Then, in L.A., I started vomiting violently, and so I got to spend the nuptials in the ER.

A colonoscopy revealed a mass in my mid-transverse colon; the colon was almost entirely obstructed. In the lexicon of diagnoses, a "mass" is way down the list of things that you want a doctor to find inside of you. Even before there had been a biopsy, the doctors were pretty sure that it was cancerous. But they wouldn't know for certain until they went in.

I will never forget the moment I woke up after my hemicolectomy in the recovery room. Josh was being consoled by Tim, the nurse, and my surgeon, Dr. D.C. He was being told that he had to take care of himself in order to take care of me. Tim asked him if he'd eaten dinner and, before Josh could answer, brought him a slice of pizza from his own dinner. Even in my anesthetized state, I knew something had to be really wrong if everybody was fussing over Josh and not me, the person who had just come out of surgery.

So when Dr. D.C.'s youthful face appeared before me, I croaked out, "Is it dire?" Based on the mood in the room, I fully expected the answer to be yes.

Instead, Dr. D.C. said, "No, it's not dire. It's very serious, but it's not dire." He went on to explain to me that he had successfully removed the tumor, but that he had found one "pea-size drop metastasis" to the peritoneum in the area above the bladder, literally a drop off the main tumor. I thought to myself, Okay that doesn't sound that bad—a pea-size drop met that was also removed—so why was Josh so upset?

I lay there in my drugged state, letting their conversations wash over me as I worked myself to greater wakefulness. Dr. D.C. said that I wouldn't remember anything that was being said that evening. Josh told him not to be so sure about that. I smiled to myself. Years of being with me had taught Josh that my mind is like a steel trap, and that, drugged or not, I don't forget anything (especially when it's something I can use against him).

I, in fact, remember a lot from that evening. In addition to the physical discomfort of having just come out of surgery, I remember thinking that the surgery must have taken way longer than the estimated two and a half hours, since it was dusk outside. I remember my brother and cousin coming to visit me in my hospital room. Most of all, though, I remember everyone throwing numbers about. One drop met. Stage IV. Six percent, 8 percent, 10 percent, 15 percent. Thirty-year-old numbers.

Because I had one metastatic spread of the main tumor to another part of my body, regardless of the size of that spread, I was thrown into the category of Stage IV. Stage IV colon cancer is associated with very low survival rates, ranging anywhere from 6 to 15 percent. Dr. D.C. repeatedly told Josh that evening that the statistics on survival rates are themselves based on thirty-year-old studies and therefore should not be relied upon.

Once I grasped that everyone was preoccupied with the numbers, I understood why Josh was so upset. Josh loves numbers. He can do complicated calculations in his head. He'd asked me at various points during our courtship, "What do you think the odds are of us getting married?" He's memorized every Super Bowl score since the beginning of the Super Bowl. He can remember that Roger Federer was down 5–3 in the second set of the third round of Wimbledon in 2009. For him, as for many people, numbers impose order in an otherwise chaotic world of randomness. And to be told that his wife had Stage IV colon cancer and therefore possibly a single-digit likelihood of living five years was understandably and especially devastating.

Josh sobbed that night and early the next morning, as he googled again and again survival rates for Stage IV colon cancer from the recliner that was doubling as his bed. The light from the iPad cast an eerie glow on his face in the darkness of my hospital room. He didn't want to discuss the statistics for fear that they would upset me, but Josh can never hide anything from me—that's one of the reasons I love him so much.

And then he was incredulous when the numbers didn't actually upset me. "So what?" I said. "Don't you *get it?*" he demanded, wanting me to understand the seriousness of the situation.

As much as Josh loves me, he cannot comprehend a fundamental truth about me simply because he hasn't lived my life. He doesn't understand that my very existence on this planet is evidence of how little numbers matter to me. Numbers mean squat. I asked him that night to go back to 1976, into the desolation and hopelessness of Communist Vietnam, and set the odds of a blind girl making it out of that unimaginable poverty, of her escaping the stigma of having a physical deformity that would make her undesirable to any man and unworthy of being any child's mother, and of her withstanding the shame of knowing that she would forever be the burden borne by a proud family that would have to care for her like an invalid for all her life.

I demanded that Josh set the odds of that little girl surviving at sea when so many grown men perished, of her gaining some sight despite years of optic nerve damage, of her achieving academic success in spite of the low family expectations stemming from immigrant ignorance, of her graduating from Harvard Law School, of her establishing a legal career at one of the most prominent international law firms in the world, and finally, of her marrying a handsome, brilliant man from the American South and then having two beautiful daughters with him. Of course, Josh couldn't set those odds.

Josh has spent many hours reading medical studies, trying to increase the likelihood of my survival. A single metastatic spread as opposed to multiple metastatic spreads yields some additional percentage points, as do my age and level of fitness, as does the fact that I have access to the best medical care in the world, as does the fact that I have a wonderful support system. According to Josh, these raise my odds of living five years to somewhere in the vicinity of 60 percent, which is to him a hell of a lot better than 6 percent.

To be honest, 60 percent doesn't sound that great to me, either. In truth, anything short of 100 percent is insufficient. But as we all know, nothing in life is 100 percent. The chance of a woman under forty having colon cancer is 0.08 percent according to a Mayo Clinic publication—Josh tells me this sort of thing because I personally don't google anything to do with statistics. That number takes into account women being afflicted with the disease for both genetic and nongenetic reasons. My tumor showed no genetic markers, which means that the likelihood of me having colon cancer is even less than 0.08 percent. My phenomenal internist told me that in his thirty-seven years of practice he has never come across a case where someone as young as I developed colon cancer for nongenetic reasons. Don't I feel so special? I had at least a 99.92 percent chance of not developing colon cancer at this point in my life, and I got it.

So numbers mean nothing. They neither provide assurance nor serve as a source of aggravation. Sure, it would have been better if my cancer were Stage I and there had been zero metastatic spread, but even when the odds are in your favor, you can still lose. For all of Josh's obsessiveness with statistical odds, he always tells me when the underdog wins the football or basketball game and defies the odds, "That's why we have to play the games."

Well, I'm here to play the game, and I choose not to live and die by what the oddsmakers say. I choose not to put faith in percentages that were assembled by some anonymous researcher looking at a bunch of impersonal data points. Instead, I choose to put faith in me, in my body, mind, and spirit, in those parts of me that are already so practiced in the art of defying the odds. Coach Taylor always told his ragtag Dillon High School Panther football team on *Friday Night Lights,* "Clear eyes, full hearts, can't lose!"

I have clear eyes and a full heart.

4

Seeing Ghosts

In the first twenty-four hours after my diagnosis, every time I thought about my children, my body would be racked with sobs unrelenting. I had often speculated about the types of women my girls would become one day. The thought of not being there to see whether Mia would indeed grow into a bright, sensitive, aloof beauty and Belle into a gregarious, charismatic spitfire made my already pained stomach hurt even more and my heart ache as nothing else I had ever experienced. The image of them crying inconsolably and in futility for me, for me to lie with them at night and kiss their boo-boos away, for someone—anyone—to love them as much and as well as I, tore my insides into a million ragged pieces.

So, for my own self-preservation, I stopped thinking about them. I told Josh to not bring them to the hospital, and when he did anyway, I kept those few visits very short. Invariably, they were unpleasant events, with Mia rushing to leave minutes after arriving because she was no doubt frightened by the tubes coming out of Mommy and with Belle being forcibly removed from my room as we were all subjected to her heart-wrenching screams. My babies became someone else's children. I knew that they were being well cared for by my parents and sister and entertained by an army of relatives. That was enough for me. I had nothing to give them during those days I spent in the hospital, as I continued to reel from the shock of the diagnosis and worked to get myself ready for and then recover from surgery.

In those early days, I could see my children only as casualties of the war I had begun fighting, a war I hadn't chosen. We were all victims of cancer, with them being the most undeserving.

Then my sweet, crazy, naughty Isabelle—this child who had grown inside my body at the same time the cancer was growing—began making me see things in a different light.

After I was discharged from the hospital, we stayed for an extra two weeks in a furnished, rented townhouse near Beverly Hills, rather than returning to New York immediately. I wanted more time in Los Angeles to follow up with doctors, recuperate, and be with family and friends I normally didn't have much opportunity to see. My parents' house was too inconveniently located on the east side. The rental was cheap and served its purpose, but it was old, dirty, and badly in need of renovations. And for better or worse, it was haunted.

Two nights after we moved in, while making our way through the usual traffic on Olympic Boulevard back to the rental, Belle declared suddenly in her babylike voice, "Mommy, I'm afraid of the dark." It was the first time my unusually articulate, not-quite two-year-old had ever talked about being afraid of the dark. But to tell the truth, I've stopped being shocked by the things that come out of her mouth, having concluded that many of her precocious statements were the results of being the younger sibling of a three-and-a-half-year-old who is pretty perceptive herself. "Belle, there are lots of lights. So you don't need to be scared of the dark," I reassured her.

Then, that night, the girls insisted that I lie down with them, especially Belle. So I lay down on the edge of the bed, with Belle next to me and Mia next to her. After a few minutes of silence, Belle sat bolt upright and said again, "Mommy, I'm afraid of the dark." Indeed, the room was dark, but it was lit by the faint glow of streetlights. "Belle, Mommy is right here. I'll keep you safe. There's nothing to be scared of. Now lie down and go to sleep!" She obediently lay down and then seconds later sat bolt upright again, looking around the room with those dark, piercing eyes of hers. "But, Mommy, I see ghosts." Now, that was definitely a first. Mia said she hadn't been talking to her sister about ghosts, and I believed her. In the past, months ago, they'd played games that involved throwing blankets over their heads and going around in broad daylight, moaning "Boo!" But for Belle to talk about ghosts and associate them with fear of the dark was a bit more than I could expect of even her. Chills ran up and down my arms.

Having just had surgery a week earlier and being keenly aware of how much closer death now seemed, I wondered if the Angel of Death was in that room, and if somehow my clairvoyant child could see him.

The next ten days passed with Belle occasionally stopping whatever she was doing in that house to stare at a spot with the look in her eyes that told us she was seeing something we couldn't see. Once, she asked whatever it was she saw, "Why did you come back?"

Another time, when our longtime babysitter put the phone to Belle's ear for her to say hi to the babysitter's sister, as she had done a dozen times before, before the sister could even speak, Belle told her, "I see a ghost in this room." After we left that house, Belle didn't fix her stare on a spot, nor did she speak of ghosts again. But I have no doubt that my child saw something in that rented house. Whether it was the Angel of Death, a guardian angel, or some other random spirit, I don't know. I do know that my Belle is special, that she has magic within her.

And after I left the hospital, Belle's behavior toward me changed. She became unusually clingy for a while. I chalked that up to the long separation of my hospital stay. The intensity of her need to be near me eventually eased. Now she will suddenly come up from behind and put her arms around my neck and hug me for a good ten seconds, which is indeed a lot of time for a two-year-old. Sometimes, she'll come up to me and plant a big wet kiss on my mouth and then throw her arms around my neck and hug me fiercely. Then I'll look into her eyes in that single second before she wants to run off, and I'll ask her, "Is Mommy going to be okay, Belle?"

"Yes," she always says.

Belle is too young to understand that Mommy is sick, yet I believe that some part of her ageless spirit understands what's going on. When Belle hugs me now, I feel as if she's giving of herself to me—her hope, her joy, her life force.

When Belle started seeing ghosts, I remembered a poem I had read in high school, "Ode on Intimations of Immortality," by the Romantic poet William Wordsworth, in which he expressed the idea that children are born "trailing clouds of glory," with the innocence, purity, and knowledge from having just come from God. It is the process of growing up, and the corrupting influence of society and life, that strips them of all their innate angelic goodness, what Wordsworth called their "hour of splendor in the grass, of glory in the flower."

And what about us adults, who are long past our moments of trailing clouds of glory and our hours of splendor in the grass, of glory in the flower? What of those of us who have been indelibly (and suddenly) scarred by our broken dreams and who might be swallowed by our own bitterness in the face of illness and impending loss? What are we to do? Wordsworth is not without advice for us:

> What though the radiance which was once so bright
> Be now for ever taken from my sight,
> Though nothing can bring back the hour
> Of splendor in the grass, of glory in the flower;
> We will grieve not, rather find
> Strength in what remains behind;
> In the primal sympathy
> Which having been must ever be;
> In the soothing thoughts that spring
> Out of human suffering;
> In the faith that looks through death,
> In years that bring the philosophic mind.

Indeed, we will grieve not for what is lost but find strength in what remains behind, through the bonds of human sympathy born of common suffering, and in our faith in something greater than we can conceive of. And no doubt, finding strength in what remains behind includes rediscovering the magic and wonder of our powerful children and letting them help us walk through our darkest hours.

5

The Warfare,
and the Weapons

An irony in all this is that before this lousy diagnosis, I was in the best shape of my life, working out five days a week. Exactly three weeks after the surgery, I was running again on the treadmill for twenty minutes. As I ran, I grew angry at the cancer. I started yelling at the cancer cells. "How dare you betray my body! How dare you threaten to take me away from my husband, babies, and all who love and need me! I will seek you out and I will destroy you!" I shrank to the size of the cancer cells and I began strangling them with my bare hands, reaching into their very DNA. Then I envisioned the chemo empowering me with a sword, with which I slashed them to a billion pieces, and then a gun. But nothing was as satisfying as crushing them with my bare hands.

Chemotherapy will start quickly, as there is reason to believe that the sooner the chemo starts the more effective it will be. I will be on a regimen called FOLFOX, which consists of three drugs, one of which—oxaliplatin—is very powerful. Common side effects: neuropathy (numbness and tingling, including extreme sensitivity to cold in the hands and feet), nausea, diarrhea, fatigue, weakened immune system, mouth sores, hair loss. Yes, *hair loss. Ugh!* So I will be shopping for a wig.

I will go in every two weeks. Oxaliplatin will be infused into me through a port (which will be implanted in my upper chest) during a two-hour period. I will then go home with a pump, through which the other two drugs will be infused into my body during the next two days.

The doctor also highly recommends switching to a plant-based diet and banning refined sugars. He says there isn't any good science to support the proposition that such a diet will reduce the risk of cancer or recurrence, but I figure it can't hurt. The most important thing the doctor told us is that there is every reason to be hopeful. My age, physical shape, the fact that all visible signs of cancer have been surgically removed, and advances in chemo are all factors working in my favor. To believe, to have faith in the face of self-doubt and uncertainty, is definitely the most difficult part of dealing with cancer. But tricks of the mind are not my forte. The life I have lived has taught me to be a somewhat ruthless realist.

6

Deals with God

I didn't grow up with any organized religion. The closest I came was going through the motions of my mother's ritualistic offerings to the Buddhist gods favored for generations in our ancestral Chinese villages, and to the spirits of my ancestors on the first and fifteenth of every lunar month. I stood before the fruit—and, on special occasions like Chinese New Year, the poached chicken, fried fish, and rice—holding the burning incense, and asked the gods and my ancestors for things like straight A's and getting into the college of my choice and, of course, health and wealth for my family.

During my great-grandmother's and grandmother's funerals, when I was ages ten and twenty, I also unthinkingly imitated the chanting, bowing, and kneeling of my parents, uncles, aunts, great-uncles, and great-aunts, all garbed in their white robes and headdresses. I didn't understand the philosophical underpinnings of the rituals, and my mother couldn't explain them to me the few times I bothered to ask. No one in our family went to temple other than maybe on Chinese New Year, and no one read any religious texts. Our quasi-religious practices were very much rooted in popular cultural and mythic traditions of village life dating back hundreds of years, and not in the esoteric teachings of Buddha and his disciples, which would have been more akin to the Judeo-Christian practices of the West. At school I couldn't help but absorb some of the teachings of those religions, since biblical allusions permeated nearly every poem, play, short story, and novel we studied in English class, and as I learned in history class, Judaism and Christianity shaped the course of Western civilization.

So I grew to believe in a little bit of everything, developing my own spiritual and philosophical approaches to life. I believe in my ancestors and that their spirits watch over me. And I believe in God, not perhaps in the image of God depicted in the Bible, but an omniscient and omnipotent being nonetheless. I think God is beyond what my little, limited human brain can fathom, but perhaps something my limitless soul can just begin to grasp in my moments of utmost clarity, moments that the Buddha would describe as the outer edges of enlightenment. For simplicity, I called all these unseen forces *God*.

I talked to (and yelled at) God a lot growing up, especially on sleepless nights, during which I angrily demanded answers to my questions, which pretty much boiled down to *Why me?* I of course have this question in common with every human who has ever lived. But we all make it our own, don't we? In my case, Why was *I* born with congenital cataracts? Why was *I* forced to live a life limited by legal blindness, forever cursed to not realize my full potential? After all, I could have been a great tennis player, a spy for the CIA, or a legendary diver like Jacques Cousteau. Why could all my cousins and friends drive and I could not? Why were all those pretty but brainless girls always surrounded by the cutest boys while I was shunned because of my thick glasses? Yes, all the things that hurt so much growing up with a visual disability became fodder for the angry tirades at God. God had a *lot* to answer for.

I listened closely for his response. I searched with my head and heart for the answers to my questions. I found them eventually, over the course of many years. I grew to embrace a belief in universal balance, something the Chinese very much believe in, as evidenced by the idea of yin and yang (e.g., man and woman, earth and sky, sun and moon, good and evil). In the karmic order of the universe, all things will return to equilibrium, and there will—indeed, there *must*—be balance.

So I made a deal with God on many of those sleepless nights. "Fine, God. If you're going to throw this crap at me, I demand to be compensated. I want the balance of my life to be restored. For everything that is bad—and you would have to agree that a visual disability of this magnitude is pretty bad—there must be a good. So, I want to name my 'good,' my compensation for all the shit that you are putting me through. I want to find the greatest love possible in this world. I want to find someone who will love me until the end of my days with an uncompromising and unparalleled love." That was the one-sided deal I struck with God again and again.

I suppose I was like most other teenage girls, my head filled with romantic notions as I read Barbara Cartland novels and Harlequin romances. My father forbade me from reading any of what he called in his broken English "I love you" books, so I hid their trashy covers behind white Chinese calendar paper, and he left me alone to dream about my Mr. Right—there are certain benefits to your parents not being able to read English. Of all the things I could have demanded as part of my bargain with God, I chose love because love was unattainable. Finding love seemed out of my control, totally dependent on timing and fate. It wasn't like scoring the perfect report card, which could be achieved through individual will and hard work. Mostly, though, I thought love to be unattainable because I believed I was unlovable. I mean, who would ever want me, as physically defective as I was? Who would ever willingly agree to be hampered by my limitations? What desirable guy would want to be forced to drive me around, read menus for me, help me down stairs, be precluded from couples sports like tennis, have his family and friends stare at the geeky girl with the thick glasses? No one, I thought.

But God accepted my deal!

He brought tall, (kind of) dark, handsome, and brilliant Josh into my life. As unlikely as it was for this Waspy good ol' boy from the South to walk unsuspectingly into the office of this immigrant girl from Vietnam with her screwed-up vision on the forty-third floor of a posh skyscraper in lower Manhattan all those years ago, the forces of the universe (a.k.a. God) made it happen. I know that many people never find the kind of love Josh and I share, a love that was tested and strengthened from the very beginning by terrifying challenges (not unlike the life-threatening challenges that face us now). From the start, I always thought Josh had the kindest and most generous heart that a human being could have (as flawed as we both are), and I tried and still do try to fiercely protect his heart from anybody and anything that threatens him. It is the least I can do for this man who loves me so abidingly, this man who makes sure my water bottle is always filled and makes me go to bed when I've fallen asleep on the couch, this man who has always read menus to me like it was the most natural thing in the world to do, this man who loves me just as I am.

But I can't protect him from cancer and all the bad stuff that is beyond my control. I can't shield him from his now constant fear of life without me. I can't take away his sense of total helplessness. I can't promise him that I will win this war. I absolutely hate what this cancer is doing to him. I hate how it makes him cry and rage and despair. I hate cancer more for what it is doing to Josh than for what it is doing to me.

Ever since the diagnosis, fear for Josh and my loved ones seems to live in every molecule of my body. Why did he sleep so much over the weekend? Could he have cancer? What about the wrist pain and indigestion he's complaining about? I look at my children with the same fears. Does Belle have brain cancer because she lost her balance that one time? Does Mia have cancer because her poop looked unusual the other day? Cancer is so insidious that it attacks your every waking thought. It's not a disease so much as it is the enemy of existence, come to turn our bodies against us. Whatever modicum of security I once felt is completely shattered. If cancer and bad shit struck once, they can and will strike again. I know it.

So I lie awake at night now with the voices in my head screaming these questions, wondering what horrible thing will happen to me and my family next. And I find myself making another deal with God, going back to my long-ago ideas about the balance between good and bad. In a world where I have no control, what choice do I have but to talk, scream, rant to, and beg of God? I tell him, "If you're going to do this shit to me again, if you're going to give me more shit to deal with in my life, fine. I can handle it. You know I can. But my husband, my children, my parents, my siblings, everyone I love—leave them alone. Dammit! *Leave them alone!* Do whatever the fuck you want with me, but don't you dare touch them!"

A woman in a support group told me that my deals with God are my form of prayer. I never thought of them that way, since I've always been so adversarial with God. But prayer or deal, he's answered and kept his end of the bargain once before. I obviously can't tell God to do anything, and there are obviously certain inevitabilities in life, like illness and death at a ripe old age, but God knows what I'm talking about, and I hope he holds up his part of the bargain this time around, too.

7

CEA, PET, MRI . . .

As previously noted, my life is numbers now. Probabilities, data points, expectancies. But when you have cancer of the gut, perhaps no number more governs your sense of well-being than the number that reflects the level of disease in your blood. Your CEA, it's called. That stands for carcinoembryonic antigen, which is a fancy term for a specific protein released by tumors, especially those found in the colon and the rectum.

When your CEA drops, the human impulse to hope makes you feel better. When your CEA rises, it can make you feel even more acutely than usual just how much your path might be starting to diverge from the path of the living.

Four months after diagnosis, my CEA was 19.8. This reflected a less than 1-point drop during the second month of chemo, whereas it had dropped 6 points during the first month. Despite everyone on the colon cancer forums and support groups saying that the CEA is a notoriously unreliable tumor marker and that it can go up during chemo, I was upset. In part, I was upset because I'm an overachiever and I like to get the A+, the perfect 100. When I had gestational diabetes, I was obsessive about getting my glucose levels to the optimal numbers through diet, exercise, and then insulin injections, and I delivered two very healthy and appropriately sized babies into this world.

But mostly, I was upset because I was convinced the CEA level not going down fast enough was suggestive of the "burden of metastatic disease." I asked to speak to the oncologist after I got these results. He took a few hours to call me back, so I texted my UCLA surgeon (who wasn't even technically my doctor anymore), and he called me within minutes. He said that obviously, we want to see the CEA lower, and that for my and Josh's peace of mind, I should have a PET scan. PET scans involve the introduction of glucose into the body combined with a radioactive tracer. Cancer cells consume the glucose, so the radioactive tracer lights up with the metabolic activity produced by the cancer.

I should pause here to mention for the benefit of other cancer patients that a good number of institutions (including Sloan Kettering) do not believe in PET scans (at least for colon cancer), on the theory that CT scans are more effective and that PET scans are more likely to produce false positives. When I went to get my third opinion, at Sloan Kettering, I was told that not only do they do solely CT scans but they do them only after treatment is completed (unless there are symptoms that would prompt earlier scanning).

My oncologist agreed with the UCLA surgeon. He told me to come in the following Monday for another CEA test, and based on those results, we would proceed with the PET scan.

For a week, I mulled over my 19.8 CEA and let it fester. It got me down. I had a few crying episodes, which is unusual for me these days. Josh played our song (Joshua Kadison's "Beautiful in My Eyes"). He had sung it to me at our wedding reception. I sobbed hysterically, thinking back on that day full of promise and glorious possibilities, when we made vows about staying together through sickness and health but had no fucking clue what was in store for us or what it's like to weather true sickness—we still don't fully understand, although we certainly understand better than we did that day. I fixated on thoughts of Josh finding comfort in the arms of another woman as he dealt with the stresses of an ailing wife, à la John Edwards. I don't think that Josh would cheat on me at this stage, but you never know what grief will do to a man.

Let me pause here to address the issue of Josh and another woman.

He and I have talked candidly about Josh remarrying if I don't make it. I affectionately call the hypothetical woman the Slutty Second Wife. I understand that if I die, Josh will need companionship and my girls will need a mother figure, and I'm okay with that. But I will state here for the record and to get this off my chest, any woman who encroaches on our relationship while I am still living will have to answer to me. And to her and the Slutty Second Wife (if she is not the same person), I promise this—if you screw with Josh and my children, either while I'm still alive or after I'm gone, if you find a way to get around my ironclad estate planning and take assets from my children into your grubby little hands, if you otherwise harm any of them, I will haunt you from the afterlife and I will hurt you.

Where were we? Oh, it was a rough week waiting for the next CEA test. When the day came, I had blood drawn at 11:30. The nurse-practitioner emailed me the results at 3:30: "Did you hear the good news? Your CEA is 1.8. It's normal!" I couldn't believe it. Normal? Is it possible to have such a dramatic drop in one week? Possible yet improbable, I suspected. I went back in to see the doctor that day. He said he was suspicious of the results and was having that blood sample re-tested. And since I was already there, I should have more blood drawn for yet another CEA reading. So I had blood drawn again at 4:30. The CEA on the retest came back at 17.8—how can a lab screw up so bad? The CEA on the second blood sample came back at 16.5. I told the doctor, yeah, great it's lower, but how can there be such a discrepancy in the CEA of the same person within five hours? He had no satisfying response—just the unreliability of CEA, and we shouldn't hang our hats on it.

Because the CEA was still elevated, I went ahead and scheduled the PET scan, right after a trip to D.C. for a colon cancer event. I had to wait through the weekend to hear the results. At least there was much distraction, with Josh's parents visiting and Mia's birthday party on Saturday. Yes, life marches on, cancer or not.

Two spots lit up on the PET scan, one to the left of the spine by the psoas muscle and one in the right pelvis. Dr. A.C. thought the spot by the psoas muscle was probably nothing. To gain further clarity, he wanted me to have an MRI of the abdomen and pelvis. Josh and I asked a series of questions: Would the surgeon have seen these spots during the surgery? *Not necessarily.* Would the CT scan performed right after the surgery have picked these spots up? *No.* Is this scan bad? *No.* Is she going to be okay, and I mean . . . *I know what you mean. Yes, I think she can be cured.*

I admire Josh for having the courage to ask that last question, and I admire the doctor for making such a statement. Nice to hear, but it honestly doesn't mean much to me. It's not that I don't have the courage to ask about being cured, but rather I think whatever the answer, it is irrelevant. Cancer is a dynamic disease. Doctors are not omniscient. An answer one day will not necessarily be the same the next day.

But all the same, I was feeling good and optimistic. The psoas muscle spot was probably nothing, and the thing in the right pelvis, if cancer, likely represented only one cancerous lymph node, but the MRI would tell us more.

For some reason, the secretary scheduled my MRI with Josh. He was anxious that I get it done right away. The only available spot was the next day at 7:45, so Josh said yes. After I completed Round 6 of chemo, he and I walked over to the MRI facility on First Avenue. Josh went home to relieve our nanny and see the girls before they went to bed. The MRI took about forty-five minutes and involved lying in a tube that made me think of coffins and being buried in the ground— more so than the PET scan, because the MRI machine is even narrower, and more confining. The only thing that was not tomblike was the constant banging and clanging of the machine, which sometimes made my entire body vibrate on the table. It also involved lots of inhaling and exhaling and holding my breath for significant periods of time. I got done a little after 9:00, took the subway, and didn't get home until after 10:00. It was a long, exhausting day.

I got the MRI results the next afternoon. The psoas muscle spot, the one that the surgeon and the oncologist had thought was probably nothing, is in fact something. There are two cancerous lymph nodes in that spot—one is necrotic (i.e., dead cancer), and the other is alive. Now you see why I don't put too much stock in doctors' prognostications.

I forwarded the MRI report to Josh. Upon review, he is "rationally optimistic." The fact is that my organs are clean, which is a good thing, and for there to be two lymph nodes involved seems like not a big deal. But you can begin to understand how absurd all this sleuthing and surmising can be. In a strange role reversal, I am not so optimistic. First of all, PET scans and MRIs cannot reliably detect growths on the peritoneum. The one tumor found (and removed) outside my colon during surgery was a drop metastasis on the peritoneum above the bladder. These recently discovered cancerous nodes are likely there.

From the beginning there has been talk about me being a good candidate for something called HIPEC surgery—shorthand for hyperthermic intraperitoneal chemotherapy—a grueling procedure that involves making a massive incision and bathing my abdominal cavity in heated chemo for ninety minutes. If it sounds equal parts sadistic and desperate, that's because it is. The procedure is also known among the cancerati as the "shake and bake." The cut is ugly, and the recovery is hard. I feel like these MRI results put me that much closer to HIPEC, and I'm not happy about it.

I've told Josh that the risk has to be sufficiently high for me to undergo HIPEC. In any event, it seems like a diagnostic laparoscopic surgery, in which a surgeon would go in to just look around, is an inevitability given the limitations of scans for detecting peritoneal growth. I also felt like I was diagnosed as Stage IV because of a technicality, due to a tiny drop metastasis to the peritoneum—a drop signifying noncirculatory invasion because it's a literal drop off the primary tumor and not cancer spreading through the lymphatic system. I felt like I was more a Stage IIIC than a Stage IV. Now these MRI results confirm that I was rightly categorized as a Stage IV, and that I have metastatic disease. All just numbers, I know, but numbers matter to some degree, no matter how much I want to deny their importance.

Because metastatic disease is almost never curable.

8

The Bliss in Making
the Journey Alone

I went through the infusion of Round 5 of chemo on a Monday in October mostly alone, with a dear friend coming at the tail end to take me home. Usually, Josh meets me at the cancer center sometime before the infusion starts, but this past Monday he had a $100+ million deal signing and he couldn't leave the office. I told him not to worry about it. I come from the world of big corporate law, so I understand how it is. $100 million isn't that much money in that world, but it's significant enough that clients have expectations. In response to his self-inflicted guilt, I reminded Josh that work, and more importantly bringing in an income to pay for health insurance and the complementary treatments not covered by health insurance, is more important than ever now. Besides, this was just one of twelve chemo treatments; it wasn't surgery; it was no big deal. Even with the cloud of cancer hanging over us, life (as distorted as life will be from now on) must go on—the children must go to school, the conference calls must take place, the bills must be paid.

Despite my nonchalance, I was sad, and Josh saw through my bravado. I had gotten used to Josh being around for my chemo days, just as he'd been around for all the days and nights when I was in the hospital and for the many weeks afterward, while I physically recovered and we together struggled to come to terms with our new reality.

So on that Monday I was alone when my blood was drawn for the usual tests. Lunch—mediocre Thai food from somewhere down on Third Avenue—I ordered and ate by myself as the oxaliplatin and leucovorin raced through my veins. I was alone when the nurse told me that my CEA results were back. I sat in my recliner by myself as the sick feeling in my stomach dissipated, and processed alone the information that it was 19.8, barely a one-point drop from last month. "Are you okay?" the nurse asked, concerned, since I'm sure the disappointment and anxiety were painted all over my face. "Yeah . . . Yeah . . . I'm fine," I weakly reassured her as a million thoughts ran through my head. Six-point drop in the first month, but only one point in the second—what does this mean? Is the chemo becoming less effective? Maybe I've deviated too much from my diet, too much sugar consumption. Maybe I'm not meditating or working out enough. Maybe the spots on my liver have become cancerous.

Josh called to check in at some point, and I told him. Maybe I shouldn't have, since he had a big conference call within minutes, but I know I would want to know if our roles were reversed. "What are the doctors saying? Get them on the phone and demand some answers!" he ordered me. He called me ten minutes later and informed me that based on his quick research we shouldn't be so concerned, that effectiveness of chemo is not necessarily reflected in the proportionate downward progression of the CEA.

I was sad that that Josh wasn't there with me, but I think it was actually good for me. Being alone reinforced something I had been feeling—and denying—for quite some time now. As terrifying as it is, battling cancer is an individual journey, and the individuality of it is what I must come to embrace. Indeed, each of us as we walk through the journey of our life does so alone. Sure, there are parents, siblings, cousins, friends, lovers, children, co-workers, and many other people who fill our lives, and sometimes their presence and chatter can make us forget that our journey is solely our own to make of as we will. But the truth is that we each enter and leave this life alone, that the experience of birth and death and all the living in between is ultimately a solitary one. While Josh may understand to some degree the distress over a CEA count that isn't dropping fast enough, he cannot know the depth and breadth of what I felt when I heard the news, nor what I feel on an ongoing basis (nor can I truly understand his emotions). A couple of weeks earlier, when the oxaliplatin brought on an episode in which I couldn't breathe while pushing Belle to school in her stroller, I endured the panic alone and found by my own will the calm within to get Belle to school and safety, and then myself to the doctor. Similarly, while I may be able to relate to some degree to other young mothers as they attempt to cope with their cancer diagnoses, our emotions are somewhat different because they have been informed by vastly different life experiences. I try to share my cancer-fighting journey with the best words I can think of to convey the complexity and nuance of the onslaught of emotions, but words have their limits. No matter how much I would like to take Josh and all who support me on this journey, I simply cannot. And I confess—I am afraid of making this journey alone.

That's hard for me to admit. I have always prided myself on being good at being alone and felt that I was one of those few people (not troubled by social disorders) who found deep joy in being alone. I thought I'd mastered the art of being alone through my solitary travels throughout the world. It's the memory of those solitary wanderings that I am now turning to in order to quell the fear I have of making this newest journey by myself.

Before I turned thirty-one I had set foot on each of the seven continents. Maybe I'm cheating, because I haven't actually been to the country of Australia yet, but I have been to New Zealand, and I think New Zealand must be part of the continent of Australia. New Zealand/Australia was the last on my list. I hiked through the South Island for two weeks in November 2006, going from one cabin to the next (New Zealand has an elaborate, although still rustic, cabin system that obviates the need for camping—a good thing as far as I'm concerned), carrying my own gear on my back (with the exception of a few pounds that others who took pity on me shouldered for the duration of the trip). Josh and I had been dating six months by then, and within three months we would be engaged. Despite our romance, Josh did not go with me to New Zealand. I didn't invite him and he didn't ask to come.

Josh understands how possessive I am about my solitary travels, how jealously I guard my experiences of discovery. I almost always went alone (meaning without anyone I knew before the start of the trip), or as alone as possible given my own physical limitations. I went to New Zealand with a nonprofit called Wilderness Inquiry, dedicated to making the outdoors accessible to people with all kinds of disabilities. I went to South Africa on safari with the same outfit in 2004. I went to Antarctica in 2005 with a group based out of Connecticut that specializes in polar expeditions without any luxury or frills. To South America, Asia, and Europe from 1995 through 2004, I generally went either as part of a study-abroad program or as a solo backpacking adventure, with, as my trusty companions, my Lonely Planet guidebooks to tell me where to sleep and eat and what sites to visit, a magnifying glass for reading the small print on maps, and binoculars for all the street signs and plane and train announcements I couldn't see.

I know there are those who think I was nuts for choosing to travel by myself and for actually liking it, even putting aside the fact of my limited vision; I know Josh must have thought this when he first met me. Eating breakfasts, lunches, and dinners of strange foods alone, wandering the great ruins of the world alone, getting lost in the growing darkness in a strange city in the hunt for that night's accommodations alone, riding on boats, buses, trains, and planes alone, with no idea of whom I would encounter in the next moment or of the future that lay ahead. You see, traveling alone was my bliss. Some people turn to mind-altering substances. Some skydive. Some play with fire. Some make fancy wedding cakes. I chose to travel the world to chase euphoria. Beyond the bliss that came from beholding the divine and breathtaking beauty of our planet's terrain and wildlife as well as the man-made creations of the geniuses who have come before, traveling alone to the seven continents represented a deeply personal journey that soothed and empowered my soul, quieting my anger and self-doubt and imbuing my spirit with a sense of unparalleled strength and independence in a way that no one and nothing else ever could.

From the moment I was old enough to think about college, I dreamed of going far away. I ended up at Williams, a little college nestled in the Berkshires in western Massachusetts, famed for its vibrant fall foliage and notorious for its frigid winters. Williams was as far away from sunny Los Angeles as I could have imagined. Even as I cried that first night in the dorm, having said a tearful goodbye to my mother and sister, I still longed to branch out. I told myself that night that despite my homesickness, I would get over it and then study abroad in my junior year. I ended up studying Chinese in college and spent my junior year in Harbin (an industrial city in northeast China known for being the first stop on the trans-Siberian railroad into Russia) and then Beijing. That year, during the months off between semesters and the periodic weeklong breaks, I hopped on all manner of transportation to far-flung provinces, listening to crowing chickens as I rode down the Yangtze River and gaping in amused horror as the door fell off the minibus taking me and a bunch of locals through the mountains of Gansu Province.

I discovered that year that traveling, and traveling alone especially, made me confront my visual disability as nothing else could. It's hard for me to explain how I see the world, in part because I don't know any other way of seeing. I can only explain my vision in clinical terms. I measure 20/200 out of my right eye with corrective lenses and 20/300 out of my left eye with corrective lenses, meaning that what a person with 20/20 vision can see at 200 or 300 feet, respectively, I need to be at 20 feet to see. In addition to that, my left eye muscle is so weak that I almost never use it. Both measurements qualify me as "legally blind," which I suppose means that I can comfortably say that I have a disability that must be accommodated in accordance with the law. These numbers don't take into account my impairment with respect to reading and seeing things close at hand. Fonts smaller than 10 points are a challenge, and even with a 10-point font, reading can be a slow process without a magnifying glass. This is how I've seen the world since I was four years old. These are the limitations that I confront on a daily basis, but nothing—absolutely nothing—makes those limitations more real, immediate, or frustrating than when I travel alone, when there's no one I know to lean on, in a strange place where I can't speak the language.

Traveling alone was the single most effective and grueling test I could put myself through, emotionally, mentally, and physically, to prove to myself that I could do as much as anyone else could. As I traipsed through the hidden back alleys of China's ancient cities and the winding medieval streets of Florence, and the unfriendly boulevards of post-Communist Budapest, searching for a youth hostel, tea house, or museum, frustrated and angry at my inability to see the numbers on buildings and read the names of businesses, I learned to control the frustration and the rage at my physical limitations. I had no choice but to find my way, for no one was there to help me. I tapped into reserves of courage and resourcefulness that I would have never known existed but for the fact that I had consciously and willingly put myself into such trying circumstances. I learned to communicate with strangers with few words, with gestures and body language. I learned to gauge the four corners of a compass by the position of the sun. I learned to stay calm, to be patient with myself, to allow myself to make wrong turns. And when I finally made it to the majesty of the Sistine Chapel and stood within the ruins of the Forum, as much as I appreciated what I was seeing, I was more grateful for my own abilities. The sense of accomplishment in knowing that I had reached my destination by my own doing was always the greatest high I could ever imagine finding—pride in my own emotional wherewithal, my own problem-solving capabilities, my own body's capacity to carry thirty pounds on my back for hours on end up and down stairs and mountains. In the greatest of ironies, traveling alone made me feel whole and complete inside; it helped to heal my anguished soul, which for so long had been obsessed with the metaphysical questions.

Part of the sense of feeling whole and complete came from the joy of meeting all the new people along the way. It was only when I traveled alone that I was truly open to meeting people and to learning everything they had to teach me about their worldview. There was also a tantalizing freedom in encountering those who knew nothing about me. Much in the same way a guy will spill his guts to a bartender, I found myself confiding in strangers about what ailed me. In these strangers' eyes, I stopped being the invalid I'd always known myself to be and I could re-create myself, transform myself into someone brave and smart and funny and engaging. I'll never forget the mysterious Swedish girl in Paris with a broken back, traveling alone in a wheelchair, with whom I shared a hostel room for one night; she told me that I was worthy of love—I know how cheesy that sounds, but that kind of sentiment is most welcome when you're traveling around the world on your own. Or the compassionate Dutchman who took the time to describe to me the details of a seascape he saw with his photographer's eyes. Or the tortured Turkish American girl who dragged me to all the techno bars in Beijing as if the loud thumping music would drown out the things that haunted each of us. All of these people whose threads of life have touched mine taught me about different ways of living, thinking, and being, and in doing so enriched my consciousness and touched my soul.

I haven't traveled alone since my trip to New Zealand. I convinced Josh to go to Egypt and Jordan for our honeymoon, and I even dragged him to China before Mia was born. We went to Puerto Rico when I was pregnant with Belle and stayed in a resort for a week. Now that I have children and am a little older, I'm not sure I would take the risks I once took to save a few bucks or have a crazy adventure I could laugh about years later. I'm out of practice when it comes to traveling alone. I've gotten used to Josh being my eyes. I've gotten used to him guiding us through airports while I deal with the children and follow him unquestioningly. I've gotten used to traveling with my little nucleus of a family and making our little trips about getting through flights without children melting down, making sure there are enough snacks to hold them over, finding child-friendly destinations where there can be no surprises and to which there can be no wrong turns. Life and priorities have changed since November 2006.

I've gotten weak and soft over the years and now I don't feel entirely ready to tackle this new phase of my life, this newest journey upon which my life hinges, which requires more bravery, strength, resourcefulness, calm, and grit than I have ever had to summon. Unlike my journey to the seven continents, this cancer-fighting journey is not one that I chose as part of some self-selected test to prove my worth. This came at me and caught me off-guard. This time I don't feel the invincibility and freedom of youth. This time I have the lives of a husband and two little girls to consider. This time the stakes are much, much higher.

Yet the bliss that can come from my cancer-fighting journey cannot be so different from the bliss I once knew traveling the world. There are extraordinary people whom I have met and whom I have yet to meet on my present course. There are lessons to be learned, resourcefulness and discipline to be cultivated, good to be done, and courage, strength, grace, resolve, and pride to be gained. I know this to be true. This is what I will remind myself when I go in alone for my first PET scan and as I listen to the doctor tell me the results. This is what I will tell myself during all the future CEA tests and chemo treatments to come. It really is okay for Josh to not be present for a chemo treatment, because his absence reminds me of the importance of being alone and honoring that solitude. All of it is part of my solitary journey, a journey that I embrace wholeheartedly and with as little fear as possible, for I know that through my wanderings I will once again find that same bliss.

9

The Secret

All families have secrets, and this was ours.

It might sound strange, but even though I wasn't told about my grandmother's order that I be killed as an infant until I was twenty-eight years old, it is something I've known from the time I was a baby. I knew it in that part of the soul that remembers all trauma even before memories can be retained by consciousness. The secret has hurt me in ways that few can imagine. Ever since my diagnosis, I've redoubled my efforts to find a lasting peace with the secret, feeling like doing so would yield hidden truths that would aid me in this fight for survival.

As my mother told me the truth about what had happened, she wept. But in her confession, I sensed the lifting of a burden long carried.

My mother had dressed me in dingy clothes that day because "it would be a waste for her to wear anything else," my grandmother had told her, glowering.

My mother did not respond—no response was required or expected—as she tried to hide her tearstained face behind the fuss of lifting me off her bed and gathering me close. With me dressed, there was nothing left to do except go. She grabbed her purse with one hand, slipped past her mother-in-law mumbling, "Goodbye, Ma," without meeting her eyes, and went down the narrow cement steps to the first floor.

Outside, my father was staring at his shoes and kicking dirt about, waiting for us to join him so we could begin our trip. It would have been like any other family trip to Da Nang to visit relatives and friends, except my sister, Lyna, and brother, Mau, were conspicuously absent, and I was conspicuously present. It was my first trip anywhere. My father had just taken the two older children to his in-laws, where they were to play with their maternal grandparents and uncles for the day. Instead of driving to Da Nang, as my parents had done so many times during the course of their seven-year marriage, we would be taking a public bus. A bus would give us anonymity, a way to get lost in the crowd and minimize the risk of relatives and friends seeing a familiar car and asking questions. On this trip, my parents were not planning to visit relatives or friends to introduce me as the latest addition to the Yip family, as would have been the expected and normal thing to do; after all, my great-grandmother had been asking to meet me now for two weeks during her periodic phone calls from Da Nang. My parents' response was pretending that the connection was bad, which was easier than telling her that they did not intend to ever introduce her to her newest great-granddaughter.

We met my father in front of the metal grille door that was open only wide enough to let a single person through. The door had not rolled open for business since South Vietnam had been "liberated" by the North Vietnamese forces, eleven months earlier. With the weight of my grandmother's stare from her second-story window on us, my parents walked silently away from the house. They walked without looking at the women who squatted on the side of the road, selling rice pancakes and rice crepes with shrimp and pork doused in pungent fermented fish sauce. They turned onto a side street and passed the two-room house of the woman who had delivered two generations of Yips into the world, my father and his brothers and my siblings, the house where my mother had given birth to me not two months earlier. And then they made another turn onto a street that lay on the outskirts of town, where the bus to Da Nang waited, its motor idling and its passengers already climbing aboard.

"One hundred dong to Da Nang per person," the bus driver told my father when we got to the door, which looked like it might soon fall off its hinges. "Fifty dong for the little one," he said as my father handed him two bills.

"But she's not even going to take up a seat," my father protested.

"Doesn't matter. Lots of people don't get a seat on this bus and they still pay full fare. You should be happy I'm letting her ride for half price," the driver said.

Not in the mood to argue with the man's reasoning, my father handed over another bill and boarded the bus, and my mother followed close behind. They were lucky to find seats at the back of the bus, because soon people were standing in the aisle and hanging out the back windows. Only when the bus could not take another single person, when a man's leg was shoved against my father's arm, did the bus finally move.

My mother was glad she was sitting. It would have been difficult to stand with a baby for two hours on the stop-and-go ride she knew this would be. Only one road connected Tam Ky and Da Nang, and its two lanes were often clogged with a steady stream of trucks, buses, cars, motorcycles, and horse- and donkey-driven carts, especially at midday. She didn't care how long it took. She would be happy if the bus broke down and they never reached their destination.

The two men sitting in front of us each lit a cigarette as they continued to talk about their plans for the day. The breeze from their window blew the smoke directly into my mother's face. She pressed my face into her chest and leaned closer to her window. The bus was passing a roadside market where people were quibbling over squawking chickens awaiting their execution, and dragon fruit, grapefruit, young green coconut, and an abundance of other fruits and vegetables in all colors of the rainbow. After the market were the lush green fields from which the bounty of the market had come. Overhead, the tropical sun cast a brilliant light, making the colors of this rain-drenched region even more alive. My mother had to squint against the assault of light and colors. Life was happening all around her. People talked, smoked, bargained, bought and sold. The world continued to move as it had always moved; it was just another ordinary day. Yet for her the world had become a dream in which she and everything she saw were not real. She had a feeling that if she tried to grab the cigarettes to toss them out the window, her hand would slip right through them as if she were a ghost, or if she got off the bus to feel the smoothness of the young coconut's skin, it would vanish in mist and the whole market would disappear with it. For the last month, she had been caught in this dreamlike state, ever since my grandmother had discovered that there was something wrong.

The only things that did feel real were the warring voices in her head. They had grown more strident with each passing day, and now on the bus they were deafening.

I can't do this!

You have to do this. There is no other way!

There must be another way. She is so beautiful, so adorable. Just look at her skin and how smooth and healthy it is. And her hair—it's so thick and shiny. Feel it! She's perfect in every other way, every single other way!

There is nothing we can do for her. Even your own parents think this must be done, not just her. You cannot let your child, whom you say you love so much, suffer through life like this.

Would her life be so bad? I would be there to take care of her. All my life, I swear.

You won't be around forever. And then what will happen to her? You already have one child who can't see right. That's enough to deal with.

I'd rather die than do this.

It was the same conversation that had been churning and churning in my mother's head since my grandmother had made her wishes known.

My mother had waited so long for me. I was to be part of her dream of having four children and a full family. Four was a nice, even number, not too many, not too few. She'd always felt that her parents' six kids had been too much, and yet she had enjoyed the noise and chaos of a full household. Lyna had come first, less than a year after the wedding, sweet and gorgeous with pale skin like our father's. As the first child and first grandchild on both sides, she had been spoiled with new sweaters and Barbie dolls and the attention of many relatives welcoming the birth of a new generation. Mau came two years later. As the first male child and the first grandson on both sides, he was especially welcomed. Everyone commented on his potato-shaped head, which they believed was a sign of incredible intelligence.

Four weeks after my birth, my grandmother had been holding me by her bedroom window. It was the first time I had been taken out of my parents' bedroom and out of my mother's sight. Consistent with Chinese traditions and superstitions, until then my mother and I had been secluded in my parents' bedroom, prohibited from bathing, required to breathe air moistened by the steam of boiling lime and lemon leaves, and compelled to follow other rituals that had been passed down from generation to generation, all to ensure that our bodies' *qi*, our life force, properly recovered from the trauma of birth, thereby reducing the risk of future organ failure and other illnesses.

Since my parents' bedroom was an internal room, the bright daylight streaming in through my grandmother's window was the first natural light that had shone on me since I had been brought home from the midwife's house hours after my birth. My grandmother, holding me on one arm with the practiced ease of one who had cared for many babies, gazed down into my face, studying me under the light, trying to determine from whom I had inherited my features. It was obvious that I had inherited my mother's dark, creamy complexion, but my large eyes were characteristic of the Yip family. She was pleased with me. Even though I was not a boy and I resembled my mother's side of the family more than my father's, I looked very healthy, with lots of meat on my bones. In fact, of her four grandchildren born thus far, I had certainly come out the biggest, a good omen in her mind considering that I was the first one born after the end of the war. She hoped that my health was a sign that things would not be as bad under Communist rule as everyone feared.

Suddenly, my grandmother's brows snapped together, her eyes narrowed as her stare intensified, and she moved closer to the window.

"Dieh!" she called to her husband, who was downstairs. After raising five sons, my grandmother had taken to calling her husband what their sons called him—Dad in Hainanese Chinese, the primary Chinese dialect spoken in my family.

My grandfather, used to his wife's many summonses, came, but not as quickly as she wanted. He stood over me, too.

"There's something wrong with her eyes. Look!" my grandmother whispered loudly to him. Her whispers were reserved for the most serious of matters, things that she did not want prying ears to hear.

My grandfather looked as he was ordered to do, and indeed he did see an odd milky whiteness in the centers of my pupils; it could have been mistaken for a reflection or trick of the light. So my grandfather held up his hand and waved it in front of my face. My eyes did not move to follow his hand; there was no change of expression, no sign that I could see his hand, waving so close and ever more fiercely.

"She's not seeing it. She's not!" My grandmother's whisper bordered on a scream. She was also now waving her hand furiously in front of my face.

"She has what her sister has. It can't be anything else," my grandfather stated in a low, matter-of-fact voice. Lyna had also been born with cataracts, although not as serious as mine.

"But Na didn't look like this at this age. She was perfect . . ." My grandmother's voice trailed off as she tried to understand what she was seeing, tried to grapple with this new reality for her and her family, tried to figure out what to do. "What are we going to do?" she asked her husband, looking desperately into his eyes. My grandfather was not one to give in to fear and panic; he believed in reason and a clear mind, the same approach he had adopted for running a successful business through decades of colonialism and civil war.

"Well, Na got better with surgery. We'll try to find her a doctor," he offered reasonably.

"What doctor? There are no doctors in Tam Ky. Na was operated on in Saigon. Saigon is days and days away from here. And even if we could get to Saigon, do you really think there are any doctors left? Na's doctor, like every other doctor, either left for Europe or America or was sent to a reeducation camp." My grandmother's tone was bitter, angry, desperate.

"We can try," my grandfather said with more hope than he felt. It was true—many of the educated had fled the country in the days before the fall of Saigon, and those who couldn't get out had been arrested and sent to camps in the countryside, where they were forced to work the land the government had confiscated from individuals and families in an effort to "reeducate" these elites in the ways of Communist ideology. Word had trickled out from those camps that their inhabitants were being overworked and underfed. There was no telling when they would be released and, when released, what condition they would be in.

"It wouldn't do any good even if we could find a doctor. The surgery in Saigon didn't fix Na's vision. Sure, she improved a little bit after the surgery, but now it's getting bad again, even though she has those thick glasses. You can tell by the way she walks around so carefully, trying to feel things. It's just a matter of time before she goes blind. Those doctors were quacks pretending they knew something so they could steal our money. And have you even thought about how dangerous it would be to operate on an infant? She would die for sure then." My grandmother spat the words as if her husband were to blame.

My grandfather sighed with exasperation. His wife was a pessimist, a chronic worrier who believed that the worst was bound to happen at every turn. But he tended to bend to her will. "We have no choice. We have to do something," he said.

My grandparents were unaware that my mother was leaning against the doorway to her bedroom next door, as if afraid to break her monthlong seclusion. She could hear the whispering, even above the squeals of Mau and Lyna, who were playing downstairs. But she already knew what my grandparents were talking about. She had seen the whiteness in my eyes days before. She had been searching for it, dreading it, knowing what it would look like, because she had seen that same whiteness creeping into my sister's eyes only a couple years before.

While living in Saigon, Lyna had begun to have trouble seeing— trying to place her toys on the table but falling short, missing the door, bumping into things. The doctor they found in the local hospital diagnosed her with cataracts, white protein growths that were clouding her vision in both eyes. He operated on the right eye first, planning to follow with surgery on the left eye several months later, but before that could happen, the Communists won the war, and then no doctors

could be found anywhere. The doctor's prognosis after the one surgery had been guarded. He said that surgery had helped, but the cataract might return to the right eye. The left eye was still untreated, its
cataract clearly visible and, to my mother, growing whiter and larger
with each passing month.

My mother told no one, not even her husband, about seeing the
cataracts in my eyes. What did it matter anyhow? Everyone would
know soon enough, and they would all blame her. I was blind and it
was her fault. She suspected that it was because of the green pills the
herbalist had told her to take during her pregnancy after she, while
helping the cook, had accidentally poured a big pot of boiling water on
her legs. She had tried to not take the medicine, but her legs had become masses of angry welts that burned like fire. Now, though, she
regretted taking the medicine; she should have just endured the pain.
Or maybe this had happened because she had eaten too many foods
with hot characteristics during her pregnancy—too many oranges,
grapefruit, mangoes—and not enough cool foods, like watermelon
and lettuce. The heat generated by those hot foods had been too much
for her baby. Or maybe it was because of her faulty genetic makeup,
which both her daughters had had the misfortune to inherit. Or maybe
the gods were simply angry with her for something she had done, and
now they were punishing her. Whatever the reason, she had failed to
protect not only me but Lyna, too; she had failed at her most basic responsibility as a mother. As the whispering went on in the next room,
my mother crawled back into her bed, careful to not make any noise
so that she could hide for just a little longer.

My grandparents summoned my mother and father to their bedroom the next evening, after the servants and the rest of the family had
gone to sleep. My mother sat on the bed beside my father as she tried
to rock me to sleep. My grandparents stood by the window. My grandmother barely looked at me, and when she did she glared. Whatever
pleasure she had felt about my presence in the world had turned to
something else—resentment, hatred even. My mother could feel her
hostility and held me tighter.

"What's going on?" my father asked innocently. My poor father,
whose hairline was already beginning to recede a little—he was truly

always the last to know. He was a good son, a good husband, a good brother, and even a good father, although a bit awkward in that role. He had always done what his parents asked of him. He had begun working for the family business at the age of sixteen, loading and un-loading heavy boxes and crates and then driving all over the country to deliver the goods for their customers. He had loved school and had wanted to go to Saigon for high school and then perhaps Taiwan for university, so he could see more of the world, but his parents insisted that there wasn't enough money, that education after a certain point was a waste of time and money; he was better off learning the family business. And so, feeling the burden of being the eldest son and prob-ably because it was the safer and easier thing to do, he gave up on his dream of learning and seeing the world. Then his mother told him he was getting too old and he had to get married and start a family. His grandmother, my great-grandmother, urged my father in that direc-tion as well, believing that his marriage and her first great-grandchildren would bring her fortune and much luck in combating her ailments. So he did what he was supposed to do and married the girl his mother chose for him. Always the dutiful son. He had no idea what was about to happen.

"Your daughter is blind," my grandmother announced to my par-ents in her loud whisper. This was not a family that minced words.

My father was silent for just a second but then regained his voice. "What do you mean she's blind? What's wrong with her?" He turned to gaze at me in denial. In the darkness of the room lit only by one bare incandescent bulb, he could see nothing wrong.

"She has the cataracts, the same thing as Na, but much more se-vere, it appears. Na can at least see with glasses. This one is not even seeing big things." My grandmother spoke with the authority of the quack doctors she so despised.

My mother knew what my father was thinking, could feel the fear even—was it genetic, was it her fault, his fault? One child to have cata-racts could be a fluke, but two? Would Mau go blind, too? She could not look at him.

My grandmother gestured to my grandfather, who had turned to stare out the window with his back to us, and then said, "Dieh and I have been thinking about what should be done, and we feel that there's no chance of fixing her eyes. There are no doctors left, and even if there were, the doctors in this country are incompetent. They could do nothing to help her. We feel that it would be best to give her something so she can sleep and never wake up. It's better to put her out of her misery, so she doesn't have to suffer needlessly."

In unison, my parents sucked in air so they would not faint from the horror of my grandmother's words, gaping up at her, searching for signs of insanity. But her dark eyes were steady and her jaw set. In her most reasonable tone, she said, "I know what I'm saying sounds drastic, but you have to think about what's best for her and what's best for this family."

My mother, so caught up in self-blame, guilt, and grief, had simply assumed that she would continue to care for me as she had cared for Lyna, hopeful that there would be a doctor, an herbalist, someone who could help now or later. She spoke for the first time, daring to challenge her mother-in-law, as she had never done before. "I can't do that to my own child. She's my flesh, my responsibility. I will care for her by myself."

My grandmother could and would punish anyone who dared to challenge her, especially a daughter-in-law who lived under her roof. "You cannot care for her by yourself, or don't you realize that? Have you forgotten that you have other children, one of whom already has vision problems? Have you thought about what her life is going to be like? *Have you?* I have! Can you imagine what it's like not to be able to see? It would be a miserable, horrible existence. I'd rather be deaf than blind. She won't be able to walk down the street by herself. She won't even be able to get around the house without bumping into things. And what about when she starts getting her period? She'll bleed all over the place, dripping like a wild bitch. And who would ever want to marry a blind girl? Who could love a blind girl? Who would voluntarily want to take care of her? *No one.* And without anyone to take care of her after you are gone, she's just going to end up on the streets begging for food like the armless and legless people you see now. Do you want your daughter to end up like that? Do you?"

My mother clutched my head and unconsciously covered my ears.

She could feel tears building up under the attack of questions and the words that felt like daggers in her stomach. She pressed her lips together, fighting the tears, because she knew that they would be viewed as a sign of hysteria and weakness.

My father spoke then. "Of course we don't want that fate for her, but don't you know that there might be some doctor somewhere who could help her? She's our blood. It just seems so wrong to do that to her." His voice was desperate, begging.

Now my grandmother turned on him. "Doctors? There will be no doctors. Don't be so stupid! You know as well as I do that come tomorrow the police may be knocking on our door and arresting you for having served in the wrong army, and you could be joining those doctors you believe in so much in the reeducation camps. And then what good will you be to this blind child of yours? Who knows if you'd even come out of there alive? Or tomorrow they could come to our house and steal the clothes off our backs, not to mention our gold if they manage to find it, just like they're doing to the other families with a penny to their name. They'll come for us soon enough. How are we supposed to take care of a blind child when we have nothing? And worse yet, a blind child who will grow up to contribute absolutely *nothing* to this family? She won't even be able to go sew or clean the house. And have you even thought about what people are going to say about us once they realize we have *this* in our family? I'll tell you what they'll say. They'll say that we are bad luck, cursed; they'll look down on us, on you and your son. Is that what you want?" Grandmother was shaking with indignation, so convinced that she knew best, incredulous that anyone would question her judgment.

There was silence. And then finally, she spoke once more, calmer now. "You two need some time to think about this and then I'm sure you will see the wisdom of what I'm suggesting. You should go to bed now."

My parents did as they were told. For the next three weeks, my grandmother pummeled them with the same impassioned assaults, until their collective will weakened, until they agreed to see the herbalist she had found, a man in Da Nang who would concoct a potion that would make me sleep forever.

By the time we came to stand before the gray concrete building where the herbalist lived, the voices in my mother's head had quieted, and in their place was a protective numbness, an armor to withstand the pain that was to come. My father, who was at his core a pessimist and a worrier like his mother, had put on his own armor since he had decided to come to Da Nang. My mother followed him up the steep stairs to the herbalist's apartment on the fourth floor. They said nothing to each other, having withdrawn into their own solitary sorrows.

My father knocked, and the door opened to reveal a man whose thinning, whitening hair suggested that he was nearing the end of his middle-aged years. My father spoke without preamble, calling him Uncle, a title of respect in Vietnamese for a man of his own father's generation. "Uncle, we were sent here by your wife. She said you would be able to help us."

The herbalist opened the door wider and stepped back to let us in. Inside was a one-room apartment, lit by a single open window and a kerosene lamp on a wooden table. In one corner was a cot, and in another a two-burner stove connected to a gas tank that sat underneath. Against the wall were shelves lined with a cornucopia of dried and drying herbs and other plants, spices, and knobby roots. Along the top shelf lay a long ivory tusk with its point blunted, perhaps by the herbalist himself when he had ground the tip and poured it into a simmering pot of thick tea to unleash the magical medicinal powers of an elephant's tusk. The room smelled of everything in nature, of trees and leaves, of roots buried in dirt, of the bones of dead animals. It smelled of decayed and decaying things and yet of life, too, for these were the herbalist's secret ingredients to improve, and sometimes to give, life.

The herbalist's wife, a woman who sold tobacco and hand-rolled cigarettes on the streets of Tam Ky, had recommended the herbalist to my grandmother. My grandmother had known her for years, but not because my grandmother smoked her cigarettes. The Tobacco Woman, with her rotting teeth and greasy hair, was well known for being closely connected to the supernatural world. The spirit of her deceased grandfather frequently visited her to guide her and advise the living souls of the community who were fortunate enough to fall within the Tobacco Woman's good graces. The Grandfather Spirit moved and spoke through a teenage boy from a nearby village who when occupied by the Grandfather Spirit would bike immediately to the Tobacco Woman's house, where he would stay for one or two days, ready to help those who sought his counsel. In exchange for allowing the Tobacco Woman to sell her wares in front of our store, my grandmother was informed with all haste by the Tobacco Woman or one of her children when the Grandfather Spirit had returned. After years of advising my grandmother by the light of an oil lamp in a one-room shack on what lottery numbers to select, which had proven more often right than wrong, the Grandfather Spirit and the Tobacco Woman had a loyal believer in my grandmother.

And now, without saying why, my grandmother had asked the Tobacco Woman for the name of a good herbalist far away from the curious eyes and ears of Tam Ky, and the Tobacco Woman had named her own husband, a man with whom she no longer lived, but a man she still believed to be a good and useful practitioner of the healing arts.

"So what can I help you with?" the herbalist asked after my parents had sat down at the table, each with a cup of tea in hand.

My father fidgeted with his faded red teacup as he said, "We were hoping that you could help us with our newborn. She can't see."

The herbalist bent over my mother and me, leaning in so he could get a better look at my eyes and pulling the lamp toward him. "Hmmm. It looks like cataracts. Surprising that it should happen in someone so young. I can give you medicine that will strengthen her eye muscles, but to tell the truth, I don't know of any medicine that will make this go away. Sometimes, we squeeze lemon juice into infected eyes, but I don't think her eyes are infected here, although it wouldn't hurt to try that, too."

"Actually . . . uh . . . we don't want you to give her medicine to make it go away because we know there isn't anything like that. We want you to give her medicine to make her not suffer so she can go someplace where she will be able to see perfectly forever," my father

clarified in a voice that was barely audible above the motorcycle en-
gines and beeping horns from the streets below.

The herbalist deliberately drew away from my mother and me
then, returning to his side of the table and his chair. "Is that really what
you want to do?" he asked.

My parents did not respond, except to look down at the cement
floor littered with bits of spices and herbs.

When the herbalist spoke again, his voice was low, too, but firm.
"You know people come to me because they're afraid of dying of cancer or they have such high blood pressure they might keel over any
second. Some women come to me because they can't get pregnant.
And I try my very best to help them all with the knowledge my father
passed on to me and the knowledge his father gave to him. I can't get
involved in the sort of dirty business that you're asking me to do. I'm
sure there are other people who can help you, but I can't. I understand
the pain you must be going through, I truly do, but I don't believe in
this sort of thing. I'm sorry."

With those words, the numbing armor around my mother began
to crack, the tears rolled down her face, and without realizing it, she
hugged me tightly and said to the herbalist, "Thank you, Uncle! Thank
you so much!" Her tears were tears of relief, of incredible joy. Her
body felt lighter, its way of celebrating this reprieve. This herbalist was
proof that there were still sane people in this world, people who
thought what she and her husband were about to do was wrong, people who would think that her mother-in-law was insane. She would be
angry when they returned with me still alive, but at least my parents
could say honestly that they had done everything they were supposed
to do and it was the herbalist who had refused to cooperate.

My father grabbed me then, hugging me for the first time in my
short life. He got up quickly and headed for the door, indicating to
my mother to follow him. He wanted to leave before the herbalist
had a chance to change his mind. My father thanked the man for his
time and rushed out the door with my mother close behind him. The
herbalist must have stared at the door long after we had gone, wondering what exactly had just happened with this odd couple who had

said they wanted one thing but acted like they wanted something else entirely.

At home in Tam Ky, Grandmother was at the door to greet us as we approached long after the sun had set. "What happened?" she demanded.

"The herbalist wouldn't do it," my father said, pushing past her with me in his arms.

"Why not? Did you offer him all the gold I gave you?" Her tone was laden with accusation. My grandmother had given my father several ounces of solid gold bars that morning, precious gold she had taken from the hiding place in the gutter behind the house, enough to compel a poor herbalist to do anything, she believed.

"No, I never got a chance. It wouldn't have mattered anyhow. The man was very firm."

"Everyone has a price. I would have been able to figure it out!" my grandmother insisted.

"Then you should have gone yourself!" my father snapped back as he turned to glare at his mother. It had been a long and exhausting day, and he just wanted it to end.

The edge in my father's voice was enough to make my grandmother back off, at least for the moment. She knew her children and when and how much to push them. But still, she could not help herself; she had to have the last word. "It doesn't matter. *I'll find another way.*"

My parents ignored her, walking up the stairs and away from my grandmother, leaving her threats for another day.

She would have found another way to kill me, too, but by then my great-grandmother had heard of her daughter-in-law's dark machinations and commanded that I be left alone: *How she was born is how she will be,* Great-Grandmother declared. And because my great-grandmother was the ultimate matriarch, her word was law and no further attempts were made to end my life. Of course, that didn't stop my grandmother from forbidding my mother to breast-feed me (which my mother tried to do in secret, but her milk soon dried up) or forbidding me from eating anything but rice gruel while my brother and sister had real sustenance (or as much sustenance as was available under the Communist regime). Because of my blindness, I was viewed as a curse on my family, doomed to a life of dependency, unmarriageability, and childlessness—and therefore worthlessness. No doubt my grandmother believed she was doing me a favor.

This secret had taken on the weight of shame, as secrets sometimes do. It was a burden that my mother could no longer bear, and so she was finally compelled to unburden herself to me. For the first twenty-eight years of my life, my attempted infanticide was an event known only to the parties involved. But on the last night of a visit home, as I sat recording my mother's voice telling the story of our family, I had a sense of what she was about to tell me. I already knew. As she spoke, I could see the scenes play out in my mind; that's why I believe that the soul remembers trauma long before the mind can retain actual memories.

It was after midnight; everyone else was long asleep, and I was to fly back to New York the next morning. My mother was spent as she came to the end of her story, and said she was telling me the truth of what had happened only because my grandmother was by then dead. She added that I was to tell no one—particularly my grandfather, father, and siblings—that I knew of the "matter." In the ensuing years, I disobeyed my mother. I recently told my siblings; I've told Josh, of course; I've told close friends; and now I'm telling the world.

One day soon, I hope to have the courage to ask my father for some answers, not in anger but in forgiveness, to gain a better understanding of the motivations of those involved, to tell him that I forgive him and my mother for their complicity. I'm just not ready yet. I've not spoken of the secret to my mother since that night, except once after my hemicolectomy, after we'd known that I had cancer for five days and I knew she was not handling it well—she was angry, fearful, guilt-ridden. I spoke to her in the privacy of my hospital room, with my sister there as moral support. "You have to tell people that I have cancer, Mom. You need to tell people so they can help you through this." No response. No surprise. My mother is a very emotionally repressed person. "Mom, you know better than anyone else how strong I am. You know better than anyone else how unlikely it was for me to be where I am today. Considering 'that matter' when I was born, you know how unlikely it is for me to even be alive, much less living the life I'm living now."

"Truly" was my mother's response, the only word she uttered during that brief conversation as she sat, bolt upright, her face set in an unreadable mask.

10

Moments of Happiness

When I was first diagnosed, I thought that I would never feel happiness in its truest, unadulterated form again. I was certain that every second in which I felt even a modicum of happiness, at seeing Mia grasp concepts like the solar system or watching Belle walk fearlessly into her first day of school, would be tarnished by cancer and that cancer's ominous presence would invariably invade every moment of my life going forward. In many ways, what I suspected would happen has happened. The joy I felt in watching my little girls dance with abandon under the flashing lights of another child's birthday party was marred by the thoughts in my head about how many future moments like this I will not be able to witness. In the midst of all that music and raucous screaming, I cried for all the things that I might never see.

Even without the cloud of cancer hanging overhead, happiness can come on unexpectedly, an elusive feeling that flits across the consciousness and is gone. Anyone who raises young children understands the oftentimes soul-crushing monotony of life's routines, of battling through fatigue to get up every morning, of rushing the kids off to school, of withstanding the stresses of the oh-so-necessary paying job, of cooking healthy dinners that will likely go uneaten by picky children, of relentlessly negotiating with the kids over when to brush teeth and what clothes to wear the next day and what treats they can have if they eat tomorrow's lunch. Before cancer, occasionally I would find flickers of the pure joy that everyone says children bring. Happiness came when Mia said something clever and funny or when Belle wrapped her little arms around me and held me like I was the most important person in the world. Joy came, too, when I spent a long weekend away with Josh or hung out with friends during a rare evening out without children. But for the most part, life before cancer, which consisted primarily of working and parenting, was plain old hard and thankless.

Don't get me wrong—I always appreciated what I had, my children's health and our comfort and well-being. I didn't need cancer to make me grateful for everything in my life. Growing up a poor immigrant and legally blind had already taught me all I ever needed to know about gratitude and appreciating life, truly. Rather, my life before cancer had settled into a routinized contentment and acceptance of the status quo, as opposed to an existence dominated by moments of happiness, defined as elevated feelings of pleasure, delight, and euphoria. After the cancer diagnosis, I simply assumed that whatever few moments of pure joy I would have would be tainted and that unadulterated happiness going forward was a total and complete impossibility.

But my assumption was wrong.

On a Thursday in the first blush of fall, I was sitting across a table from my former obstetrician, Dr. C., at a nondescript eatery buried in the dinginess of lower Manhattan. We were sharing a late lunch of spinach, brown rice, and roasted vegetables, which was incidentally entirely anticancer and antidiabetes compliant. We were in the midst of a conversation that had been going on for two hours, one that had begun in the lobby of my gym, where Dr. C. had met me, one that would go on for another two hours as we walked through the streets of Chinatown. Our conversation was about everything. We first talked about my cancer diagnosis, how it had come to be, potential medical causes, my CEA level, possible future surgeries, the merits of going outside New York City for additional treatment, her belief in my ability to beat this cancer because, in her words, there is nothing typical about me. We talked about Dr. C.'s recent trip to Uganda, the reverse culture shock she was experiencing, and her plans for the future.

It was in the middle of this conversation that I blurted out, completely unbidden, "You know what? I'm really, *really* happy right now."

Even I was a little surprised at this declaration. How is it possible to have Stage IV colon cancer and feel for even a second, much less the many moments of that afternoon, the kind of carefree joy that would prompt me to make such a statement?

Much of it had to do with Dr. C. herself. Indeed, there is nothing about Dr. C. that is remotely typical, either. She had returned only two days earlier from six months in Uganda, volunteering at a hospital with 550 beds to which people would travel for days and at which patients would sell a cow to pay for surgery. She showed me pictures of the hospital nursery, which was nothing more than a table where babies lay, with their mothers' blankets wrapped around them as the only proof of maternity (for there were no ID bracelets). She told me crazy stories about how she had sawed off the gangrened arm of a pregnant woman who had been gored by a bull and how she had to remove a mother's dead fetus as well as the remnants of her ruptured uterus after a failed home delivery, all under harrowing conditions where anesthesia, electricity, resources, and expertise were in short supply. Dr. C. had shut down her practice of twenty-five years, during which it felt like she had delivered nearly every child in Tribeca, in order to go to Uganda as part of a commitment to serve underserved areas at home and abroad, a commitment she had made when graduating from medical school.

When she closed her practice and left for Uganda, I doubted that I would ever see her again, because it was clear that she had no intention of returning to New York. I had written her an email a couple weeks earlier to let her know about my diagnosis, not entirely expecting her to respond. It was only upon her return to the United States that she read my news and contacted me immediately to convey her shock. I asked to see her then, told her in fact that I absolutely needed to see her.

Dr. C. has, since the day I met her, always made me feel safe. She diagnosed me with gestational diabetes during both pregnancies and forced me to keep (and email to her) a daily food journal that recorded everything I consumed as well as my blood sugar levels at specific times each day. Just as she did for all her other patients, she showed up at the hospital the moment I arrived (as opposed to the end of labor, as so many other obstetricians do). She, not a nurse, held me when the anesthesiologists administered the epidurals. She coached me through the pain of labor and delivery, and was essential to the healthy arrivals of Mia and Belle into this world. As a solo practitioner, she did not take a single vacation in the twenty-five years prior to closing her practice, and in return for her devotion to her patients, her patients have an un-wavering loyalty to her.

I know my friends who are also former patients would have loved the opportunity to spend an afternoon with Dr. C. The truth is that the only reason Dr. C. took an afternoon out of her limited time in New York to talk to me was that, as unlikely as it is, I have cancer. If she were still practicing and I didn't have cancer, we would never have talked about our lives in such an honest and open manner, entering the realm of a friendship that I hope will endure for years to come. It is a privilege to have been cared for by Dr. C. It is even more of a privilege to know and be inspired by such a good and courageous human being, who wants to, and indeed does, make a true difference in the lives of everyone she touches. In spending time with Dr. C., I was happy be-cause I didn't expect to be. I was happy because out of cancer had come this new relationship and a new understanding about another human being who had already been so important to me and my family. I was happy because through knowing and talking to her I felt in those moments an enrichment of my life and soul.

The sudden prospect of a shortened life and imminent death seems to have the power to do that. Relationships are accelerated—acquaintances can become intimates in an afternoon. Because there is no time to waste, and what is more important than intimacy?

I've been thinking quite a bit about the moments when I've been the happiest in my life. You might expect me to say it was the moment I married Josh, or the moment I held each of my squirming daughters for the first time. Alas, no—sorry, Josh and Mia and Belle. As honest as

I am, I have to admit that marriage and bringing forth life, while filled with joy, were too fraught with anxiety to be truly and purely happy moments. I wondered, subconsciously anyway, as I stood by Josh's side in my pretty white dress, whether our relationship would endure. As I learned to hold my firstborn against my body, I wondered if I were going to break her fragile body or otherwise fail her as a mother. It would have been naïve and arrogant of me not to have those thoughts then.

No, when I think of the happiest moments of my life, free from anxiety and worry, I think of the time I sat atop a hillside with three Tibetan monks in the distant province of Gansu, China, at age nineteen, listening to the haunting chants from the monastery below. I think of sitting in a Zodiac on Thanksgiving Day 2005, making my way through white, green, and blue water toward the Antarctic coast under the brightest sky and sun I'd ever seen, to meet hundreds of wild penguins. I think of riding on a bicycle rickshaw along the country roads of Bangladesh too narrow for a car, under a star-filled sky with hundreds of fireflies lighting our path. These were the most euphoric moments of my life, moments when I was at peace, however briefly, when I had no worries about my past or my future, when I had traveled alone long and often difficult distances to reach my destination, when I felt gratitude in the breathtaking beauty I was so privileged to behold, when I felt like my soul was expanding to encompass a rare and even divine part of the human experience, to see and feel places of such extraordinary natural wonder that they must surely have been touched by the hand of God.

As shocking as it may seem, cancer has brought me moments of happiness. My moment of happiness with Dr. C. wasn't so different from the moments of happiness I'd experienced during my travels before cancer. While cancer has the capacity to tarnish my happy moments with my children, to taint them with doubts about the future, cancer also has an incredible ability to strip away the ugliness and the things that don't matter and to put everything in a perspective as bracingly clear as that Antarctic sky. With Dr. C., I forgot about the dreariness of that restaurant. I forgot about the uncertainty of my future. Instead, cancer gave me an ability to focus on the present, to really listen to everything Dr. C. told me, to enjoy and marvel at her stories and her as a human being and our human connection. And because cancer forces me and others to refocus on what matters, what I have found, as with Dr. C., are people coming forward to strengthen and reestablish old relationships or establish new ones—former doctors, high school classmates, fellow parents, distant friends, people I've never even met. It is these relationships in my life, a life that for better or for worse is so defined by cancer now, that matter to me most these days, that make me truly happy. It is in these relationships that I am finding the breathtaking beauty, peace, and divinity I once ascribed only to my solitary wanderings.

11

An Adventure with
the Chinese Medicine Man

In early October, a friend whose mother is facing a rare, lethal form of breast cancer strongly recommended that I go see Dr. G.W., an expert in dispensing herbs to treat cancer and other ailments as part of traditional Chinese medicine practices. Initially I was skeptical, in part because my beloved internist is dead-set against herbal supplements—he wrote an entire chapter in a medical textbook about the untold risks associated with taking them. I had also assumed that my oncologist was opposed to traditional Chinese medicine as a form of either alternative or complementary treatment (as most oncologists seem to be), although we'd never discussed the topic specifically. The fear is of course that, in the absence of clinical studies to show otherwise, the herbs might interfere with chemo treatments and have other negative ramifications, resulting in the promotion of cancer growth and additional unpleasant consequences.

But my friend was insistent, and her recommendation was impassioned; so I looked into Dr. G.W. His credentials were impressive—PhD from Harvard some thirty-five years ago, professorships at various prestigious institutions, years of cancer research at Sloan Kettering, and numerous legitimate-sounding papers and presentations on herbal research. Plus, the breast cancer community online raves about Dr. G.W. Breast cancer is his specialty, but according to his website, he does have experience in other cancers, including colon cancer. The clincher, though, was that my friend's mother's doctors spoke glowingly of him, and that my own oncologist, while he doesn't know Dr. G.W., was comfortable with me taking herbal supplements, so long as he approved in advance the herbs being used. The fact that my blood is being tested all the time also provides him (and me) comfort; if the herbs caused negative effects, they would show up in my blood.

More irrationally, I've been emboldened by Siddhartha Mukherjee's *The Emperor of All Maladies,* a beautiful and brilliant work that chronicles the history of cancer and the work of daring doctors and researchers and their patients who heroically—many said stupidly at the time—risked their professional careers and lives to develop revolutionary drugs to fight off this scourge that has plagued the human race since our beginning. If those brave souls could take such risks with potent, untested chemicals, I could roll the dice with traditional Chinese medicine, which after all has been around for thousands of years and is a part of my noble Chinese heritage.

So I sent Dr. G.W. an email, and he called me. He told me to meet him on the corner of Forty-seventh and Broadway in Astoria, Queens, in front of the Rite Aid. Odd, but okay. For those not from New York, Queens is a borough that no one ventures into unless one lives there. Think of Vince, Eric, Drama, and Turtle of *Entourage* fame, who escaped the obscurity of Queens for the glamour and glitz of Los Angeles. Think of Carrie, Samantha, and Charlotte of *Sex and the City,* who cringed in horror at the idea of visiting Miranda in Brooklyn (gasp!); Brooklyn was bad enough for those sophisticated Manhattanites; forget about Queens; Carrie Bradshaw's treasured Manolo Blahniks would never have touched a sidewalk in Queens. While Brooklyn offers the charm of elegant nineteenth-century brownstones and gorgeous Prospect Park (the outer boroughs' response to Manhattan's Central Park), Queens has little to offer in terms of aesthetics, with its streets characterized by squat and square redbrick buildings. I've been to Queens only a few times, because my sister lives in Astoria, and I've tasted on even fewer occasions the amazing ethnic food that only Queens offers.

The point is that making my way to Queens to meet the Chinese medicine man on some strange street corner was an adventure. My parents (who were visiting from L.A.) insisted on going with me, and they dragged my sister along, too. The four of us stood on the corner of Forty-seventh and Broadway in front of the one-story building that houses a Rite Aid—my brother was the only one missing out on all the fun. I called Dr. G.W. and told him I had arrived at our designated meeting spot; he said he would be there in five minutes. My parents kept asking me, "Aren't we going to his office? Why are we standing here?" I couldn't answer their questions, as I was starting to wonder myself whether this guy was legit. I stood waiting with my little entourage and giggled with my sister over the ludicrousness of the situation—here I am standing on a street corner with cancer cells floating around in my body, waiting for an alleged doctor to give me mysterious herbs. I felt like I should be wearing dark glasses and a trench coat. My parents didn't seem to find the situation very amusing. I told them to lighten up.

As I waited, I remembered some of the bizarre adventures I'd had in China. The Chinese (as do people in most other parts of the world) have an unorthodox and frequently sketchy way of doing things, especially when viewed from the perspective of Westerners, for whom order and the rule of law are dominant forces. On multiple occasions, I nodded to a man muttering "CD? DVD?" on the streets near the famed Silk Alley in Beijing, where fake and nonfake American- and European-branded clothes, shoes, and accessories could be had for serious bargain prices. I'd then followed the man to an abandoned building where I handed over very little money in exchange for a lot of pirated CDs and DVDs. Back in the mid-1990s, it seemed like any transaction that promised little money for great reward involved some man or woman leading you from a public place to an abandoned back office or stairwell where hotel rooms could be booked, tickets purchased, and currencies exchanged; it always reeked of illicitness. And I loved it all! The risk taking, the unknown, and the strangeness got my heart pumping and my blood flowing with excitement, amusement, and a real joy for life.

I suppose waiting for Dr. G.W. wasn't all that different. Why couldn't a miracle cure be found on the street in front of the Rite Aid?

I was curious, entertained, and excited—and somewhat wary. When my father saw a lone diminutive man in a floral shirt carrying a black satchel ambling down Forty-seventh Street, he said in a tone dripping with sarcasm, "That must be him. Really looks like a Harvard-trained doctor." Indeed, it was Dr. G.W. "Who are all these people?" Dr. G.W. asked me suspiciously after we confirmed one another's identity. He accepted without comment my response and allowed my entourage to trail behind us as we walked.

We walked back down Broadway to a little café. I ordered sandwiches for myself and my parents, thereby giving us the right to use the café for a medical consultation. We climbed up to the second floor, which was empty of people. I sat with Dr. G.W. at one table, and my parents and sister sat one table over, openly eavesdropping on our conversation, which lasted well over an hour.

Despite the oddity of it all, I like Dr. G.W. I do think he's legit. He said that he could have met me in his office at a prominent hospital in Manhattan, but that would have required my information to be logged in to a computer system and would have severely limited him in the advice he could give me. According to Dr. G.W., the medical establishment distrusts traditional Chinese medicine. While there are those who support it (like people at his hospital), that support is kept quiet, for fear of liability. Because there are thousands of herbs and infinite herb combinations, and because little money is invested in testing the use of those herbs in treating cancer and other diseases, doctors and hospitals are paralyzed when it comes to traditional Chinese medicine. Dr. G.W. pointed to the all-powerful and richly endowed Sloan Kettering as the worst of all in their conservative views.

After reviewing my most recent blood test results, feeling my pulse, looking at my tongue, and just generally observing me, Dr. G.W. felt that the classification of my cancer as Stage IV was a mere "technicality," and that I am strong and exhibiting minimal side effects from the chemo. He certainly had a hopeful and very reassuring manner, which I really appreciated and needed desperately that day. The objective while I am in treatment is to minimize the chemo side effects, detox my body, and boost my immune system (i.e., maintain my blood and platelet counts at normal levels to obviate the need for painful shots).

Once I'm out of treatment (if we get there), the focus will shift to preventing recurrence.

I'd half expected him to pull out a bunch of herbs from his black satchel like Mary Poppins would pull out a lamp from her purse, but alas, that did not happen. He gave me instructions to go to an herbal pharmacy in Chinatown (the only one he trusts, as they've been around for forty years and are known for sourcing high-quality herbs). When I was little, my mother would bring home mysterious brown herbs wrapped in pink butcher paper, dump them in a pot, and cook them for hours. Then she'd force down the bitter black tea resulting from that brew. Fortunately, it's thirty years later, and now herbal pharmacies have machines that brew teas and package them into vacuum pouches that are easy to use. I am grateful to not have to brew teas for hours as my mother did, because if I'd had to, I might not have ever embarked on this little adventure.

The day after our meeting, Dr. G.W. sent me the list of herbs that would make up my tea:

Poria
Dioscorea
Atractylodes
Codonopsis
Astragalus
Cinnamon twig
Mulberry twig
Perilla leaf
Ophiopogon tuber
Schisandra
Peony
Ligustrum
Achyranthes
Eucommia bark
Cornus
Lycium fruit
Chih-ko
Magnolia bark

Lo hon fruit

Tangerine peel

I forwarded the list to my oncologist. He approved. I told Dr. G.W. to place the order with the herbal pharmacy, and I went to pick up the tea. Amid the open-air markets of fruits and vegetables and smelly fish and the restaurants with the roasted ducks and chickens hanging in their windows sits the uncrowded herbal pharmacy. The store looks as reputable and clean as a store in New York's Chinatown can be, with glass display cases under fluorescent lights filled with creams, ointments, and oils, and shelves lined with hundreds of giant glass jars containing things like black jujubes, honeyed dates, lo han guo, and all the other manner of fruit, tree bark, leaves, fungi, roots, and derivatives thereof that could possibly be in the world. One of the teenagers working behind the counter went into the back room to retrieve my freshly brewed teas, all neatly packed in four-ounce clear plastic pouches. The tea was so newly made that it was almost too hot to handle. I authorized a $150 charge on my credit card for a sixteen-day supply and walked out the door. (Credit card acceptance in Chinatown is also a good sign of legitimacy.) Dr. G.W. will reassess the herbal formula at the end of that period to determine if there are any necessary adjustments. My job is to drink the stuff twice a day and to keep him informed via email about how my body is reacting.

Bottoms up!

2014

12

The Surly Bonds of Earth

An interesting quirk of having a disease is that most of your friends from diagnosis on also have the same disease. Which means that pretty soon, your friends start to die.

The first week of 2014 brought this part of the experience home, vividly. I celebrated my thirty-eighth birthday, observed the six-month anniversary of my diagnosis, and learned of the cancer-related deaths of two individuals and the impending death of another. One of the dead was a veritable celebrity in the colorectal cancer community, and the other I had known and worked with shortly before my own diagnosis.

John was a partner at my law firm, a distinguished-looking man in his mid-fifties who, despite having lived all over the world practicing law, hadn't managed to rid himself of his midwestern accent. I didn't know him as well as I knew many other partners of the firm, but I was briefly assigned to work on a transaction with him only last June, just as I was first experiencing symptoms. He was one of those partners who was always involved, who actually read the documents and called to check on the status of various aspects of the deal. Of course, I was going on vacation to L.A. in early July, so John decided to replace me with another associate.

Little did either of us know then that deadly tumors were thriving in both of our bodies. In early December, I learned that John had just been diagnosed with brain cancer and the prognosis was grim. And then, two months later, he was dead. It took me two months just to begin processing the fact that I had cancer. He didn't even have a chance to put up a fight.

John passed away the day after Gloria died of colon cancer–related complications. I didn't know Gloria personally, but I read her entire blog, which chronicled her three-and-a-half-year battle, when I was first diagnosed. She had a loud voice in the colorectal cancer community, since she'd started her own nonprofit to raise money to find a cure. Diagnosed at age twenty-eight with aggressive Stage IV disease that involved widespread metastases, she was given one year to live, two at most. She was known for her warrior attitude, relentless positivity, and even enthusiasm for fighting the disease—so seemingly fearless, positive, and enthusiastic was she that she never really wrote of her fears or sadness, and instead seemed almost happy about the "opportunity" cancer presented in her life—which to me verged on the delusional.

To those of us who followed her progress, it certainly seemed that until the day she died she truly believed that she would beat the cancer, that the cancer had picked the wrong person, that, in her words, "Cancer, your time is up."

She had been quiet publicly about her decline in part because people believed that by virtue of her unyielding ferocity in the face of this deadly disease, she would indeed somehow win her war. The fact that her body had succumbed alarmed many who drew inspiration from her and felt that if the fierce WunderGlo (her chosen nickname) couldn't overcome, how could they?

And then there is lovely Kathryn, a tall, fifty-something Minnesotan who has lived long past her initial prognosis. She's been a dedicated source of support and information for others and a devout builder of the colorectal cancer community—she was the one who found me and brought me into Colontown (a support group on Facebook). I've met Kathryn but don't know her well at all, unless you count the real intimacy of her writing on Colontown. I admire her brave decision to stop all chemo a few months ago, and I admire how she is spending the last days of her life on this earth, at home in hospice care, with her family and friends, even as her body is slowly being starved to death because a tumor is obstructing the path into her stomach. Even as she is constantly vomiting what little water she can ingest, she makes the effort to inform everyone as she has always done of the details of her medical condition and her mental state, which is calm and gracefully accepting of her coming death. In so doing, she is demystifying the process of dying, helping all of us who will also one day die be less afraid.

In so doing, she is giving those of us who love her a chance to bid her farewell, to say our piece.

Those of us who face cancer, any type of cancer, are prone to use the metaphor and language of war to describe the way we deal with our disease; I myself have described chemo as the most powerful weapon in my arsenal, the receipt of bad news as a defeat in one battle among many, and all of my supporters as my army. In many respects, it's an appropriate and useful metaphor because it lends a visual image to an often long and arduous process with an uncertain outcome in which the mind and body are brutalized; it fires up passion and gets the adrenaline flowing and can push one to keep enduring. But what happens when the body can no longer tolerate further treatment? What happens when death is the outcome of the war and not life? People hate to think that Kathryn, Gloria, and John have ultimately "lost" their personal wars against cancer, and yet there is no denying that reality; John and Gloria are gone, and Kathryn will soon follow.

As I've said before, battling cancer occurs in not just the physical realm, but also the nonphysical realm, where the mind and spirit are challenged to find the will to keep fighting, to feel happiness despite the sadness, to find light amid the darkness, to laugh through the fear, to live with abandon and joy under the specter of death. I hope that no matter how difficult the physical war becomes for me and no matter how I may struggle through the nonphysical war, I will always confront my disease with the same kind of courage, honesty, grace, and acceptance that Kathryn has exhibited, she who learned so much about her disease and its treatments, both established and experimental; she who shared that knowledge as no other; she who recognized when chemo was compromising the quality of her life during the little time she had remaining; she who chose to accept with dignity the overwhelming power of the cancer in her body.

Cancer is a force of nature that acts within the human body, just as the winds and rains from a hurricane are forces of nature that act on the earth. We are so small, insignificant, and powerless in the face of those unleashed forces in spite of the marvels of shelter and modern medicine. There comes a time when one must admit that powerlessness and evacuate ahead of the deadly hurricane, rather than remain behind and make some kind of empty symbolic gesture of "fuck you." Similarly, there comes a time when one must recognize the futility of continuing the personal physical fight against cancer, when chemo is no longer a desirable option, when one should begin the process of saying goodbye and understand that death is not the enemy, but merely the next part of life. Determining that time is a deliberation that each of us must make with her own heart and soul. This is what Kathryn has done; she respects the force of nature acting on her body and has no delusions about somehow still overcoming; she made the cogent decision to evacuate ahead of the hurricane. To me, she has won her war against cancer so valiantly fought in the nonphysical realm.

Yet another dying friend, C, just posted on Four Corners (a subgroup of Colontown that is exclusively for those of us with Stage IV colorectal cancer, where we can freely and safely say the things that would terrify those who live with a lower-stage cancer) about what it was like for her—as per the family therapist's suggestion—to sit in the next room as her husband and sister-in-law told her children that treatment was no longer working and that their mother was going to die from this disease. What it was like to hear her children's cries and not be able to comfort them, for that heartbreaking task had to be left to their future caregivers.

These are the times in life when we feel almost more than we are capable of feeling. These are the moments when—paradoxically, as we are closest to death—we are most painfully and vividly alive.

13

The Crossroads of the World

A crossroads is a place where multiple roads converge, and is a point at which a decision needs to be made about what road to take as one continues on the journey. Which way to go? When my final day of chemo arrived, on January 13, it certainly felt like a crossroads, a decision point where scans would soon follow and Josh, my doctor, and I would have to decide what to do next. So somehow it felt right that I should end up at Times Square, known as it is (ostentatiously) as the Crossroads of the World.

January 13 felt like a momentous day—Cousin N, who is like a sister to me, had flown from Los Angeles the day before to be with me for the last session and to spend the week; Cousin C, who is also like a sister to me and who lives in Connecticut, left her young children for twenty-four hours (something she hadn't done in four years) to sleep over the night before so she could come with me to chemo as well. My actual sister, Lyna (who lives in New York City), also came to spend the night—Lyna and Cousin N slept on the full-size air mattress, and Cousin C took the couch.

As we like to remind each other often in a half-joking way (especially when one seems to have become spoiled by her soft life), no matter how Americanized we have become, we can never forget that we came to this country on a sinking boat from Vietnam and should have no problems sleeping on couches, air mattresses, and floors; a carpeted floor covered by a flat cotton sheet was where we slept often as children, with not even the padding of a sleeping bag—what did a bunch of Vietnamese refugees know about sleeping bags?

That night, Josh stayed home with Mia and Belle, and we four Yip girls went out to a dinner of fancy Asian fusion fare at a restaurant in the South Slope, opened by a *Top Chef* winner, laughing and gossiping just as we used to when we were little girls, except now we gossiped and complained about our aging Chinese parents, husbands, children, money, careers (or the sudden disappearance thereof), and all the stuff of ever-impending middle-aged adulthood. It felt so comfortable and yet poignant; how sad that it took something like my last session of chemotherapy for advanced colon cancer to bring us together again without boyfriends and husbands and children, in a way we hadn't been in more than twenty years.

While in the cab to the restaurant, as we all stared and giggled at the scantily dressed girls freezing their butts off hurrying to a Jay-Z concert, I had one of those strange passing sensations in which I felt removed from my body and observed this current scene of my life as if I were watching a play on a stage, speculating about whether my character would suffer some tragic ending in the play's denouement. I wondered if one day, perhaps not so far away, my sisters would reunite again without me, and if they would remember that particular moment of laughter. And where would I be?

Cancer has made me hold these precious scenes of my life against my heart like they're my very own children; that's how much I cherish them. And while those scenes can make me feel a longing I've never known, they also make me feel an unparalleled joy and appreciation.

During dinner, Cousin N casually mentioned that she needed to meet one of her "reps" at Times Square at 10:30 the next morning. Cousin N is in advertising; she buys and plans media for a major motion picture studio, meaning she decides where to buy and how to use advertising space (e.g., TV and radio commercials, magazine ads, posters in subway stations, et cetera) for blockbusters and every other kind of movie this studio produces. She has become a big muckety-muck, overseeing large teams of young assistants who do her bidding. "No problem," I said. "Whatever you need to do for your job." Chemo was scheduled for 12:30, so we would have plenty of time.

The next morning, after Cousins N and C accompanied me to drop Mia off at school—my sister had left early for work—we made our way to Forty-seventh Street and Broadway and stood in front of the red steps that are just south of the famous TKTS booth, where tourists line up for hours to buy half-price tickets for Broadway shows. Times Square is normally a place I avoid like the plague, filled with tourists who walk too slowly and too many flashing lights; it's a place that can overwhelm in seconds. But it was early on a Monday morning, so it was relatively sane, devoid of the usual mob and the oversize Elmo, Dora, and other characters clamoring for their photos to be taken in exchange for five bucks, and devoid of other crazies like the Naked Cowboy (who goes around even in the dead of winter with nothing on but cowboy boots, underwear, a cowboy hat, and a guitar). Cousin N was talking to Joel, her rep, a few feet away while I was engaged in a heated conversation with Cousin C about how she should make sure her children are appropriately exposed to their Chinese cultural heritage.

Suddenly, my best friend, S.J., showed up. What a coincidence! I went on and on to her about how really small New York City is despite being home to 8 million souls. Just then, I saw Josh walking toward me, and I was equally amazed to see him. "Oh my God!" I shouted. "Times Square really is the crossroads of the world!" And then I saw my sister approaching. Before I could open my mouth to demand to know what was going on, Cousin N told me to turn around. "Look!" she said.

Please note that when you tell a legally blind person—or at least this legally blind person—to look!, it engenders a certain panic. Add to that the Times Square environment, where there is an infinite number of things to look at and even more panic, and you fear you won't see what everyone wants you to see. But even I couldn't miss the giant screen featuring an enormous picture of me when I turned around.

There it was, along with, in letters as big as me: CONGRATS JULIE, ON YOUR LAST CHEMO SESSION TODAY! WE LOVE YOU! The picture was up for a long time, four minutes maybe. And then Cousin N announced, "But wait, there's more!" More? I wasn't sure I could handle more! Joel gave the thumbs-up to the invisible people looking down at us from somewhere above, and the picture disappeared and the live camera feed went on and there I was on the digital billboard with Josh by my side, along with Cousin N, Cousin C, Sister Lyna, S.J., and of course Joel. And then the people who couldn't resist the allure of seeing themselves on the big screen in Times Square came swarming in, like moths to a flame. The camera zoomed in on me and Josh, and I covered my face in embarrassment. While Josh might look like a politician on camera with his polished wave, I am no politician's wife, uncomfortable underneath the weight of all that attention.

Cousin N and Joel had orchestrated the whole thing. Joel and his company sell time on the digital billboards in Times Square. N told him what was happening with me, and he was apparently so moved that he insisted on doing something special. I can only imagine how much advertising revenue Joel's company sacrificed in order to put up an ad about a cancer patient on her last day of chemo. I wrapped my arms around him, and much to my surprise, I wept uncontrollably into his wool coat.

You see, I am not so old that I have forgotten the deeply rooted feelings of being unwanted, and so I still don't know what to do with kindness. This gesture from my cousin and her friend was moving enough, but the fact that it was a visual gesture, and on such a grand scale, well, that made my knees buckle.

My mother had my siblings go to Chinese school to learn Mandarin Chinese after regular school, but never me. *You won't be able to read the Chinese characters,* she told me. Fifth Uncle took my siblings and cousins to see *Star Wars: Return of the Jedi* in the theater, but not me. "Why don't I get to go?" I asked my sister. *Because you might not be able to see the screen,* she said. (Translation: no one wants to waste money on you.) Once when I was nine, Cousins N and C and my sister all got to go to San Francisco to visit Fourth Uncle and I didn't get to go. Why? I asked my mother. *Because you can't see like everyone else, and no one will take care of you* was her response. From a young age, I felt marginalized; I felt defective because I was told through actions and words that I *was* defective.

So I spent many years proving that I could see well enough to go to the movies, to travel the world on my own, to study Chinese (I lived in China during my junior year in college, and became fluent). I did it all for many reasons, but mostly it was to prove my own worth to myself and my family. I felt as if I had to prove myself into existence every day, because my existence was a proposition that had early on been very much in doubt. At some point, when I had accomplished all that I had dreamed of accomplishing and indeed gotten married and had children and done those things that everyone once said I wouldn't be able to do, I began to feel self-worth and love from within as well as from without. But to a large degree, I could never let go of those feelings of being unwanted and unloved, so ingrained had they been in me from such a tender age.

I'm pretty sure that feelings of insecurity are nearly universal. I see the insecurity already in my children, even though they have had the benefit of nurturing teachers and (I'd like to think) nurturing parents. I'm always amazed at how the beautiful and intelligent never feel quite beautiful or intelligent enough, how people constantly agonize over not being thin enough or charming enough. And all of these things matter—beauty, intelligence, weight, and hundreds of other criteria by which people judge themselves—because these are the characteristics people select to determine whether they're indeed desirable and lovable.

Ultimately, we all have a constant need to be accepted and loved in this world, to feel connected to the communities represented by networks of family, friends, colleagues, church, and the other groups that surround us. To belong, to matter to someone, to feel comfort. It's almost as if the fear of being unloved is part of our genetic makeup, or maybe it is deeper even than that, and is endemic to being born human on a tiny rock floating through infinity. That realization is enough to make even the least self-aware person a little insecure about what it all means, and what our role in this passion play might be. Ironically and rather unexpectedly, cancer has proven to be most effective in chasing away my insecurities, allowing me to shed almost completely those old and painful feelings of unlovability.

How funny that one of the two greatest challenges of my life—my visual disability—should make me feel so unloved, and that the other greatest challenge of my life—this cancer—should rectify that, resoundingly.

I am humbled. That unwanted and unworthy little girl is truly baffled by all these acts of love.

14

Hope

In March, on the eve of my HIPEC surgery, I wanted to write about hope. It's a word that is bandied about so frequently when you have cancer. "You cannot give up hope," Josh has told me many times. "There's always hope," more than one cancer survivor has told me. People have recommended to me a book (which I've read) called *The Anatomy of Hope*, one oncologist's account of how important it is to maintain a realistic hope, sprinkled with tales of patients defeating cancer against all odds. This fuzzy concept of hope, this feeling that something desirable can be attained, is so prevalent in the world of cancer that it takes on a holy quality that people embrace purely on the basis of faith: like, if you have it, it will sustain you through your darkest hours, and maybe even cure you. Because the word is invoked so often, hope can also feel like a lie. After all, how can you say there is always hope when clearly at some point death is imminent—where is the hope then?

It is to my mother's stories of life in Vietnam and our escape that I've turned often in the last eight months as I've examined the value of hope. Her stories reveal the mercurial nature of hope; it is like a fire in our souls, sometimes flickering weakly, like the flame of a single candle in the night, and sometimes raging mightily, casting a warm and brilliant light of limitless possibilities.

My thirty-year-old mother was one of the many who had lived through years of civil war and one of the many who watched with envy as the few Vietnamese who had ties to the Americans, or guts, or luck, or money, or some combination of these things managed to flee the country. Riding behind my father on his moped through the busy streets of Saigon in the final days of the South, my mother witnessed firsthand how truly lucky some were.

One of her most vivid memories was this tableau: an American soldier pulling on the arm of a pretty Vietnamese girl, clearly urging her to come with him; an older woman who no doubt was the girl's mother pulling on her other arm, obviously begging her to stay. It was a tug-of-war that symbolized the opposing forces of America and Vietnam, old and new, brightness and darkness, success and failure, even life and death. Finally tiring of the game, the soldier with his easy strength picked up both women in his arms, dumped them in his jeep, and drove off into the evening sun.

My mother longed to go after them, to inhabit the glamorous and rich world of Marilyn Monroe and Jackie Kennedy that she'd glimpsed in the occasional American movie. More important, she wanted to leave Vietnam in order to find better medical care for my older sister, whose vision was also impaired. How to do it exactly, she had no idea. Escape, much less escape to America, was a dream, a fantasy, a hope so impossible that my mother pushed it away to the recesses of her mind, and instead focused on surviving under the new regime. Yet, dim as it was, the hope of a different and better life was born in my mother on the day the soldier tossed those women into his car, you're-coming-with-me style.

Obviously, my mother's far-fetched hope came to pass. The poverty became so extreme that hundreds of thousands were prepared to risk their lives at sea, fleeing in the dead of night. As more and more people escaped, and letters and pictures arrived from France, Australia, and America proving that a new life was indeed possible, my mother's impatience with her circumstances grew and grew and grew. But unsanctioned escape was almost exclusively for the single and young, who had easy mobility, who could move about in the dark of night in order to snag the one or two spots left on a fishing boat leaving on the spur of a moment. Despite my mother's building hope, there was still no way to manage the evacuation of an entire family that included my seventy-nine-year-old great-grandmother. Ultimately, geopolitical forces played out in our favor as cooling relations between Vietnam and China caused the new Vietnamese government to "invite" all ethnic Chinese to leave—a mild form of ethnic cleansing—subject of course to adequate payments in gold and the transfer of all property to the state. So in February 1979, my family—at least fifty people—boarded different fishing boats, bound for Hong Kong and Macau.

The rickety fishing boat I was in measured roughly fifty-four by twelve feet and carried three hundred people packed against one another. The journey to Hong Kong lasted a month and included eleven days on the open seas with little food and water. We were lucky because our boat did not sink, as so many others did. We were lucky because we were not forced to engage in cannibalism, as some refugees were. Less than a year after we arrived in Hong Kong, the United States Catholic Church sponsored my immediate family's emigration to the United States, providing the funds for our Pan Am flight from Hong Kong to San Francisco. On November 30, 1979, my mother's long-standing hopes were realized when we set foot on American soil. I was three years old.

I once asked my mother whether she was afraid when she sat on that precarious fishing boat, at the mercy of the sea gods and countless other gods who controlled her and her family's destiny. I wondered as she sat there for days on end, looking out on the vast expanse of ocean, what she envisioned in her heart and mind, what she hoped for in those moments of absolute terror when she and everyone else were violently seasick, when she and her children were hungry and had no idea when refuge would be found. Did she dream of Jackie Kennedy? Did she have images of American streets paved with gold? Did the hope embodied in such images keep her going through the darkest moments of her journey?

"I wasn't afraid because I had no expectations at that point," she said. "I didn't really think. When I thought about the future, whether it was the next day, the next month, or the next year, it was just blank whiteness. There was nothing beyond that moment, that second even." In order to get through the ordeal, my mother essentially banned hope from her consciousness so she wouldn't be incapacitated by fear. She stopped thinking and moved instinctively, living one second at a time. I think that's what people call survival mode.

In this war against cancer, I, too, have found the need to go into survival mode, to envision a future of blank whiteness. Each time my heart is broken in this war, out of a primal sense of self-preservation, I vow that I will never allow myself to feel that kind of debilitating disappointment, devastation, and pain again. I can't bear it, I tell myself. It is in the darkest moments with cancer and as I recover from the latest defeat that I say "Fuck hope" and forbid my mind and heart from creating happy visions of a distant future that is entirely unlikely. I'm afraid to hope. And so in those moments, I don't cling to hope to sustain me as so many say I should. Rather, I reject it.

Hope is a funny thing, though. It seems to have a life and will of its own; it is irrepressible, its very existence inextricably tied to our spirit, its flame, no matter how weak, not extinguishable. After disappointing CEA results, and after a weekend of feeling like it was futile to fight this war, I came to grips with the latest setback and started being able to see beyond that day and that week and then that month. Soon, I decided that I realistically had eight good years left, that I could see eight years out when my children will be ten and twelve, and that I was going to focus on compressing a lot of living into those eight years and whatever I got on top of that would just be sweet icing.

But no more dreaming of retiring with Josh; no more imagining holding grandchildren in my arms. From now on, it was about establishing a concrete, specific, and entirely achievable goal, and if I made it to that goal, then I would think about the next attainable goal.

I would parry hope, and defy it to toy with me again.

Josh and others thought I was overreacting, prematurely giving up hope because of one CEA result. In truth, it was my coping mechanism. I needed to toughen up; I needed to change my expectations if I was going to get through the inevitable future setbacks; otherwise, I would be destroyed emotionally.

This was me—turning to face the killing force inside me. I wanted to see it clearly. My life has been far too stark and difficult to let myself

slip into denial now. Denial is first cousin to hope. But all good things—
the beautiful, impossible life Josh and I have created, for instance—
came to be only by facing hard truths consciously. Such realism had
served me well, and as enticing as magical thinking can be, now was
not the time to give in to its seductions.

Then we went to see Dr. D.L., the HIPEC surgeon, and Josh asked
a question that I would have never been able to bring myself to ask:
Could HIPEC be a cure?

And, with those words spoken, I could feel the flame of hope grow
a little brighter inside me, in spite of the vow I had made to myself.
And since then, sometimes thoughts and dreams of a life beyond the
eight-year mark have crept into my head, unbidden. People tell me
they know that HIPEC will cure me, that I will be one of the lucky
ones. I don't want to believe them because I can't bear the thought of
more heartbreak, but a tiny part of me hopes they are right.

Until cancer happened to me, I never understood the vicissitudes
of hope; I never understood the joy, terror, and despair it could bring;
nor did I understand its incredible resilience. The best analogy I can
come up with for those who have yet to live with cancer is the undying
search for an enduring and romantic love, something that is nearly
universal to the human experience. Before Josh, there were a few guys
in my life. But there were one or two who truly broke my heart, creating the kind of ugly blubbering and depression that embarrasses me
now when I think of it.

Nothing hurts quite as much as young love, when it seemed like
my entire sense of self-worth was tied to these guys who so brutally
rejected me, leaving me feeling utterly unlovable. Each time, I swore
that I was done with men, that I didn't want to put my heart at risk
again, that I didn't need a man to make me happy. And each time, time
would make me forget the pain. Time and experience taught me new
strength and courage, giving me the fortitude or the foolishness to put
my heart at risk again and again—until I finally met Josh.

I think I will always oscillate between embracing and rejecting
hope. I think I will always live somewhere in between today and eight
years and forty years from now. But what I do know about hope is that
it is an everlasting and indelible part of my spirit; it is there even when

I feel hopeless, a perpetual flame. I have felt its faint warmth even in my darkest moments, even as I've sought to squash it. I know the flame, however weak or strong, will burn so long as I live. And near the end of my days, when it is clear that more life is not possible, my hope will evolve into something else, into hope for my children, hope for the human race, hope for my soul.

15

I Am Lost

I can really cook.

In late spring of 2014, I took to posting pictures of my culinary achievements on Facebook—short rib lasagna rolls, chicken pot pie, turkey soup with kale and loads of other vegetables. Those photos symbolize an ostensible return to "normalcy," for, before cancer, I loved to cook and had a little problem with buying too much kitchen stuff. Some people have an addiction to acquiring clothes and shoes; I had an addiction to buying high-end cookware, kitchen gadgets, and cookbooks. The best Christmas presents Josh ever got me were my 7.25-quart Le Creuset Dutch oven and a ninety-five-dollar instant digital thermometer. For months after my diagnosis, I stopped cooking. The neuropathy from the first chemo regimen made cooking annoying and even painful. But more critically, I had lost all pleasure in food, convinced against all rationality that everything I ate would make the cancer grow. Ironically, during my most recent hospital stay, when I was denied all food for four and a half days so my bowels could rest to clear the small bowel obstruction, I obsessively watched PBS cooking shows on my iPad and drooled over David Chang's fancy ramen noodles as I lay in bed weak from hunger. I vowed then that I would never shun food again.

I also posted on Facebook a photo of our new car, a small SUV, another stab at normalcy. It's a considerable expense for something that we will use only two or three times a month, but we decided that it was a necessary part of moving forward with our lives, so that we could go hiking, pick apples in the fall, and explore cute towns on the weekends.

But behind those photos and the rush of activity, behind the smiles and my seemingly upbeat statements to everyone about how I was so glad not to be in the hospital, to be walking upright and to not be in pain, behind the pose, I was broken emotionally, more broken than I can remember ever being. Oftentimes, choosing fabric, researching cars, cooking a new recipe, all these ostensibly life-affirming acts felt like me clinging to a piece of wood in the vast ocean, acts of grave desperation that would only put off for a time the unavoidable truth and great inevitability, the truth being that I have cancer and the inevitability being that I will eventually die from that cancer.

I took my girls to two birthday parties one balmy weekend in May. The first was for one of Belle's friends from school. None of the parents in Belle's class know about my diagnosis. So when I stood there making nice with the birthday girl's mother, a tall, beautiful woman living in a beautiful glass building on the edge of Prospect Park, everything made more beautiful by the glorious blue of the spring day, I wanted to scream at her, *"I have fucking Stage IV colon cancer! Do you have any fucking clue?"* The second was a joint birthday party for three of Mia's classmates held at the carousel in Brooklyn Bridge Park with spectacular views of the towering skyscrapers in lower Manhattan as the backdrop. The parents in Mia's class know about my diagnosis, so I was left to answer awkward questions about how I'm doing from people who may or may not care, so happily ensconced are they in the unblemished perfection of their own lives, or, if they do care, are afraid to pry. "Oh, fine. Just hanging in there," I say vaguely. I want to scream at all of them, too: *"This is so fucking unfair! I didn't deserve this. My children didn't deserve this!"* But I keep these and millions of other bitter, angry, and unkind thoughts to myself. I don't break social decorum, and I keep my fake smile firmly plastered on my face.

Unconsciously, I use the thoughts to form a wall around myself, a wall with which to keep the person I love most in this world—my poor, beleaguered, hurt, exhausted, terrified Josh—out. I lash out at him in anger; I push him away; I don't tell him what's really on my mind; the thoughts are too involved, too depressing, too sad, too imbued with guilt. I feel guilty for marrying Josh and ruining his life. I was the last girl Josh or anyone from his family expected him to marry when he was ten, fifteen, eighteen, or even twenty-five. Let's be honest. He was born and raised in the true South, in the mountains of South Carolina, where the Confederate flag still flies in the state's capital. He went to an Episcopal parochial school from kindergarten through twelfth grade and then the University of South Carolina for undergraduate and law schools. No one would have dreamed in a million years that he would marry a legally blind Chinese American girl born in Vietnam, raised in Los Angeles with the occasional ritualistic Buddhist tradition, and educated in the distasteful liberal and Yankee institutions of the Northeast. I can't help but think that if he'd married a blond, Christian, southern debutante, then I and my illness would never have ruined his life. I know: if I hadn't met Josh, then Belle and Mia would not be here, and they are our greatest joys. No one says that guilt is rational.

Josh is angry, too, angrier than I am. He lashes out at me, too, even though his anger is directed at the gross injustice of all of this, at the unseen forces that shape our lives. Why is this happening to us? he wants to know. He feels an irrational guilt, too. He thinks that he should have done something to save me, that he should have known cancer was growing inside me. The guilt eats at him like a parasite. He goes about his life, almost as if everything is normal, working his long hours and thinking about convoluted investment structures that comply with the Internal Revenue Code, putting on his dapper suits to meet clients and close deals, in a sick, twisted manner finding some escape in the pressures of work. The hard things for him are the memories of our life before cancer, especially now, as we near the one-year anniversary of the diagnosis. The NBA playoffs this year trigger thoughts of last year's playoffs and how we were so utterly and stupidly clueless then. My return to cooking reminds him of what he calls our "Halcyon days," those innocent days before cancer, when our lives were carefree and happy. But as for me, what's hardest of all for him is operating under the strain of trying to be normal.

He agreed that buying a car would be a good idea, and as he sat with Lenny, our car salesman, making small talk, he wondered what would happen if he yelled, "My wife is fucking dying!" And then we smiled pleasantly and drove out of the dealership with Lenny being none the wiser . . .

16

A Nightmare

Today, July 7, 2014, is the one-year anniversary of my cancer diagnosis. I don't wake up in the middle of the night screaming, but the memories do come back to me unbidden, sometimes triggered by being in a particular place or by what someone says or by nothing at all; sometimes, they feel like waking nightmares. They play out in my mind's eye like a Greek tragedy in which I am watching myself with dread, knowing that I, the protagonist, will meet a terrible fate even as I go on so innocently and stupidly believing that my pain was just IBS or some other obscure intestinal disorder, but certainly not cancer. As the tragic hero of my own play, I will be brought down by my fatal flaw, my hubris, which would have me believe that I am young and strong (with my five-times-a-week workout schedule) and that I am immune from cancer. But as a member of the audience, I know what's coming, and I want to scream at my alter ego, warn her so that her fate might be something other than what it already is.

I remember feeling sick that first Friday in June after eating my favorite yogurt, and so began four weeks of bloating, belching, cramping, nausea, loud gurgling noises in my stomach, and mental and physical listlessness that would come and go with ever-increasing frequency and intensity. I remember asking Josh the following week to pick up Gas-X for me on his way home from work per the doctor's orders because it was probably just irritable bowel syndrome. I remember on multiple occasions lying in bed after my nanny had left for the day, dazed, and Josh coming home from work late to find the children were still running around in all their craziness because I simply couldn't manage to put them to bed.

I had just finished reading *French Kids Eat Everything* and was determined to get my kids to eat everything, too, by, among other things, sitting down with them to dinner every night; I remember how I just couldn't eat as I sat slumped on the couch. I remember lying in the bathtub on the Tuesday evening exactly a week before going to Los Angeles for the wedding and family reunion, hoping that the hot water would ease the pain, and then throwing up and not having the energy to finish the memo I had to write for work about a hugely important Delaware court decision. Later, my internist told me I should have called him then, that I should have gone to the ER then; so many "should-haves." I remember going to see him two days later and how concerned he was because my symptoms had gotten worse since my first visit, two and a half weeks earlier, and how he had me see a gastroenterologist immediately because I was supposed to go on vacation the next evening, and how he thought that was a bad idea considering how sick I was, and how the gastroenterologist ran blood tests and scheduled me for an ultrasound the next morning, and how the gastroenterologist told me that afternoon that my blood work seemed fine and nothing seemed amiss on the ultrasound so he was giving me the okay to travel. But if I was still having issues upon my return, he would have to perform an endoscopy and a colonoscopy.

I remember us driving to the Hudson River Valley that evening to hunt for our future weekend home and battling through the discomfort all through that weekend as the severe constipation really set in. I remember getting on the plane to Los Angeles the following Tuesday, July 2, in a zombielike state and somehow making it through that flight with two young children and then the awful midafternoon traffic to get to my parents' house in Monterey Park (a predominantly Chinese suburb east of Los Angeles) and then eating my dad's marinated ribs (one of my favorite dishes) even though I hadn't pooped normally in who knew how long and lying in bed afterward, exhausted and in pain. I remember my mother coming home from work that night and being horrified at how pale I was—"green," she said in Vietnamese— and at how thin I had gotten in the less than two months since she'd last seen me; I wondered later whether mothers have a sixth sense about their children. I remember . . . I remember . . .

The next day, Wednesday, July 3, Josh and I went to the Staples in the next town over to fax some papers to our Realtor—we had bid on a house, had accepted the seller's counteroffer, and were about to sign the contract. While Josh was trying to figure out how to work the fax machine, I asked a cashier for a plastic bag, found a corner where I hoped no one would see me, and threw up a warm, yellowish-brown substance into the bag. By evening, I was vomiting water. I called the doctors in New York covering for my internist and gastroenterologist (it was a holiday weekend, after all); they both told me to go to the ER. Josh drove me to Garfield Medical Center, a few blocks from my parents' house, where I found a bunch of elderly Chinese people waiting to be seen. "I'm not going to wait," I told Josh, "it will go away," and we went for a walk around the block instead, hoping that that would make this bout ease. I wanted to hold on until I returned to New York, in less than a week. I should have waited that night, but maybe a part of me knew that if I checked in to the ER, I wouldn't be leaving for a while, and I didn't want to miss the big family reunion that was going to happen at my brother's house the next day.

On the Fourth of July, we all congregated at my brother's Mediterranean-style house in the hills of Palos Verdes Estates, where you can see the Pacific Ocean from the backyard. I was gratified to see my girls play in the inflatable pool and run around with their first and second cousins. It was what I had wanted. I was so happy to see my parents, siblings, cousins, and uncles and aunts all together, laughing and talking in the many languages that I grew up with. For the briefest of moments, I could relive the most joyous parts of my childhood.

By 4:00 A.M. on the day of the wedding, I couldn't take it anymore. I woke up my seventy-year-old father and asked him to drive me to the hospital. I didn't wake Josh because I wanted to spare him whatever this was for a little longer, so he could have a few more hours of sleep; I intuitively knew he would need all the sleep he could get to deal with whatever awaited us that day and in the days to come.

There was no one in the ER at Garfield Medical Center this time, which was fortunate because I was in so much pain I couldn't even sit up straight when the triage nurse assessed my condition and admitted me. I'll never forget my incredible relief when the morphine hit my system; I could understand why people would rob and kill for narcotics. The ER attending told me that he'd seen what appeared to be an obstruction on my CT scan so he was going to admit me to the hospital. I remember thinking, Well, at least a physical problem can be identified. Even at that point, cancer didn't enter my mind.

Had I thought it might be cancer, I would not have gone to the ER at Garfield Medical Center, a hospital that serves a large, indigent, and underinsured immigrant population, filled with poorly educated and dubiously trained doctors. The surgeon assigned to my case, an idiot whose English was so accented I struggled to understand him—you know it must be pretty bad for me not to be able to understand a Chinese person's accented English—and whose speech patterns and movements reminded me of a drunk, reviewed my X-rays and told me he saw nothing and that I would just have to wait for the obstruction to pass on its own while on bowel rest. The gastroenterologist assigned to my case, Dr. Tran, the only competent doctor there, didn't agree with that approach; he was actually intent on discovering the nature of the obstruction. He ordered a CT scan with contrast for a better-quality image for 9:00 that evening, and planned to do a colonoscopy at 9:00 the next morning—July 7.

Josh and my sister came to see me after the CT scan, sneaking in long after visiting hours had ended in their fancy attire to tell me about the wedding, show me videos of the girls dancing, and let me know everyone was very concerned. Then Josh told me he loved me, told me to get some rest and that he'd see me in the morning, before they took me in for the colonoscopy. That was how the last day of my innocent old life ended.

The next morning I was taken to a room where Dr. Tran waited to do my colonoscopy. Just as I fell into that twilight state reserved for most colonoscopies, I saw Dr. Tran's fuzzy face and heard him say, "I saw a mass in your colon on the CT scans." Then I knew.

I woke from the anesthesia as I was being wheeled back into my room. Josh was waiting for me. The destroyed look on his face confirmed what I already knew. He was trying so hard to act calm and not cry, but the devastation was obvious. Then he said the words and showed me a copy of the colonoscopy report. "They found a mass that is suspicious for cancer . . . seventy-five to ninety-nine percent obstruction of your transverse colon." Of course, Dr. Tran had said we wouldn't know for certain until the biopsy results came back, but Josh and I knew that there was no need to wait for biopsy results, that words like "suspicious" are loaded in the medical world. We cried together in confusion, shock, horror, and fear.

Suddenly, my father and sister were there. They said nothing, but their faces reflected what I felt. My mother was at home taking care of the girls—oh my God, what would happen to my sweet, beautiful little girls? Then my brother, who had dropped everything upon hearing the news and driven the forty-five minutes to Monterey Park, was there at my bedside, hugging me and crying. I could see all the grays in his coarse, straight hair as he laid his head on me. I had stopped crying by then as I held his hand—I couldn't remember ever holding his hand before. When had he grown up into a man and a father? When had I grown up into a woman and a mother? How was it that we were dealing with matters of life and death already—my life and death, to be precise? Here was the person who had taught me how to hold a baseball bat as he sought to transform me into the little brother he never had. And there was my sister, who had always taken care of me, whether it was driving me to buy clothes as a teenager or navigating us through the streets of some foreign place in our many travels together. And there was my father, who had always shamelessly admitted to all that I was his youngest and most treasured child, the only person who could legitimately contend with Josh over who loved me best. And of course, there was Josh, my lover, my best friend, my soul mate, the father of my children.

In that hospital room, with the exception of my mother and little girls, were the people I loved most in the world. It was a surreal scene, something from my worst dream, except I'd never dreamed this night-mare of the people closest to me in this life crying over me like I was already dead. I wanted to pinch myself awake and find myself back in New York living the life I knew and loved, but the pain in my hard and distended abdomen reminded me constantly that this was all too real and that this was a living nightmare to which there was no foreseeable end.

17

The Hand of God

I follow no institutionalized religion and have no patience for pros-
elytizing, but I do have faith in a higher power—most of the time,
anyhow. In my elusive moments of faith, when I am alone and still
and no one asks me to verbalize or justify that faith, I know with a
certainty that I could never explain that the hand of God has touched
my life.

Even as the memories of that period of diagnosis continue to trau-
matize me, I also recall that time with a certain fondness. It was a magical period full of beauty and incomparable love; and it is that sense of
magic and wonder that also resonates for me of providence.

Even as I and my immediate family were trying to process the fact
that I had cancer and fighting through the paralyzing shock in my tiny
half of the hospital room that Sunday morning of July 7—I don't think
we had quite made it to the point of thinking about what had to happen next. For I think it was literally minutes after Josh had handed me
the colonoscopy report and my brother was still sitting by my bedside—my cellphone rang. A caller from New York with a phone number that was vaguely familiar. Automatically, I answered, "Hello?"

"This is Dr. F. We spoke the other day when I advised you to go to
the ER. I'm just calling to check in and see what happened," the voice
on the other end said. It was the doctor covering for my internist, Dr.

N.L., over the Fourth of July weekend, calling me on a Sunday and minutes after I had received this devastating news. Did he have a sixth sense that something had happened?

I was just so happy to hear a medical voice from "home," at least the place I considered my adult home, where my life was, where my trusted doctors were. My response was immediate, even if it was somewhat panicky and tearful. "I'm so glad you called, Dr. F. I just received the results of my colonoscopy. I have a mass blocking seventy-five to ninety-nine percent of my transverse colon, and it's suspicious for cancer!"

The briefest moment of silence, and then Dr. F. said, "I'll call you right back." My phone rang again a moment later. "I just spoke to Dr. N.L., and we both agree that you need to get out of that hospital and get yourself to a reputable facility in Los Angeles and you need to find a colorectal surgeon immediately."

A colorectal surgeon? What was a colorectal surgeon? I'd never ever heard the word "colorectal" in my life. And how the hell was I going to find a colorectal surgeon, and how was I going to get to a reputable facility? I was hooked up to an IV that was giving me food and pain and antinausea meds, and I was severely uncomfortable with a stomach that made me look like I was four months pregnant. It wasn't as if I could just walk out of the hospital. All those thoughts hit my brain at once. I knew one thing for certain, though, even in my shocked state—there was no way in hell the incoherent surgeon at Garfield Medical Center who had said that he'd seen nothing in my X-rays and that the blockage would just clear on its own was ever going to touch me. I hated him and that hospital and I wanted to leave immediately, but not to another facility in Los Angeles. I wanted to go back to New York, to doctors I knew. "Coming back to New York for surgery is not a good idea," Dr. F. stated firmly when I told him I wanted to go home. Dr. F. and Dr. N.L. knew of no colorectal surgeons in Los Angeles. I would have to find one myself.

True, I had grown up in Los Angeles, but I had left twenty years earlier. I knew the big hospitals were Cedars-Sinai—that's where all the celebrities seemed to go—and UCLA, but I certainly knew no doctors at either place. So Josh and my siblings started alerting my cousins, first to let them know what was happening, and then to ask them for any leads on colorectal surgeons. No doubt my mother, true to traditional Chinese values, would have been horrified that we were publicizing the shameful details of my diagnosis, but it's a good thing we did, because within the hour Cousin C called me—she had also come back to Los Angeles for the wedding.

Cousin C, with whom I grew up and who is like a sister to me, wasted no time with the emotional stuff—there would be plenty of time for that later. She was all business with me on the phone, as was I. We are Chinese. We are immigrants. Our ancestors escaped poverty and war by fleeing to Vietnam, and we and our parents did the same by fleeing to America, "on a sinking boat no less," as my cousin N likes to say. Pragmatism flows through our veins. Cousin C lives in Westport, Connecticut, now, but for years she lived in Maplewood, New Jersey, next to a renowned gastroenterologist whose practice is in Manhattan. She hadn't been in touch with him for years, but she would email him to see if he had any recommendations. Paolo was his name. I never learned what his last name was. Paolo responded promptly to Cousin C's email even though they hadn't communicated in so long, and it was Sunday of the Fourth of July weekend.

Yes, he wrote, one of his actor patients had gotten surgery last year from a Dr. James Y. at UCLA, and he'd been quite happy with the result. Could Cousin C please provide him with Josh's cellphone number and he would reach out to Dr. Y.?

A couple hours later, while Josh was in the car with my brother, on their way to pick up some lunch and considering some unpromising leads for a surgeon, Josh's phone rang. "Hi, Josh. This is Jim. Paolo told me about your situation. How can I help you?" A top surgeon at UCLA calling Josh on his cellphone on a Sunday during a holiday weekend and being so incredibly friendly and helpful—it absolutely defied all of our preconceived notions about arrogant, aloof surgeons. Dr. Y. told Josh that he would operate immediately, before seeing any biopsy results, because in almost all cases, something like this was cancer. He told Josh he would be glad to take me as a patient and that he would serve as the accepting doctor in the hospital transfer process. Josh and I were relieved and ecstatic. This was the first step in me getting out of that hellhole of a hospital.

A worsening obstruction with increasing pain and nausea, combined with the frantic desperation of knowing that I had a malignant growth inside me, made the few hours that had elapsed feel like days and weeks, and so we quickly moved (or at least we tried to quickly move) on to the next step in the process—getting through the hospital and insurance company bureaucracy to effect the hospital-to-hospital transfer, and by "we" I really mean Josh, because he was the only one capable of dealing with such matters at that point. Josh is not one of those people who likes dealing with the details of life (e.g., paying bills, buying soap, planning vacations, arranging for the fixing of broken appliances). He also hates talking on the phone, whether to order a food delivery or resolve the faulty cable. When there's an issue of any sort, I'm the one who calls to complain and demand and take care of it. During the more than twenty-four hours it would take for me to be transferred, I would witness a new side to my husband as he extended himself to do what did not come naturally to him. He would call and harass the various parties involved as we waited and waited and waited—the staff at Garfield Medical Center, the staff at UCLA, the insurance company—as UCLA sought to assure itself that my insurance company (unfamiliar to West Coast medical providers) would pay the bills.

I was lying there forlornly late that Sunday afternoon, starting to realize that a transfer that day was looking less and less likely given the nonresponsiveness of my insurance company, when my room phone rang. It was someone calling from UCLA for me. The guy on the other end wanted to verify my identity. "Mrs. Yip-Williams, our records indicate that the name associated with your social security number is Ly Thanh Diep . . . our records indicate that your address is 911 West College Street, Los Angeles, CA . . . our records indicate that your phone number is (213) 250–0580." My name had at one point indeed been Ly Thanh Diep, and my address and phone number thirty-three years ago had been exactly as the man said. Thirty-three years ago I had received my eye surgeries at UCLA, the surgeries that would give me sight. That was the only possible reason why this man was reciting this ancient information about me. And yet somehow, realizing that I was going back to the place where I had received my first surgery ever, which had in a certain respect saved my life, after all these years made me feel like I was coming full circle, like there was a certain comforting rightness about what had happened and what was about to happen, like the nudge of God's hand.

Josh was on the phone with the insurance company at 5:00 A.M. local time the next day, trying valiantly to push the bureaucracy along. With the start of regular business hours and the return of a full staff, my insurance company moved much more quickly. By late morning, we received word that UCLA had financially cleared me for the transfer—a further hurdle crossed. However, there was to be yet another.

There were no available beds at UCLA and there likely wouldn't be a bed until Wednesday or Thursday, we were told. I was horrified—Wednesday or Thursday? I felt certain with the worsening pain in my gut that I would be dead by then. We briefly considered ripping the IVs out of my arm so that Josh could drive me to the ER at UCLA—that would surely get us a bed. Reason prevailed, however, as that strategy held a certain amount of medical risk and uncertainty, not to mention uncontrolled pain and nausea, In desperation, Josh called Dr. Y. on his cellphone and begged him for help. Dr. Y. made a few phone calls and informed us that there were in fact twenty-eight people ahead of me in line for a bed at UCLA Ronald Reagan, and that he could do nothing about moving me up in that line, in spite of my desperate physical condition. However, UCLA Santa Monica—a branch of the main facility—had a "favorable" bed situation; Dr. Y. himself did not operate at Santa Monica, but he would get me to the best surgeon at Santa Monica. My financial clearance would be good for either UCLA facility, so there would be no further delay in that regard. Josh and I were desperate—yes, whatever; we need to get out of here!

I could feel myself closer to death with every minute that I remained at Garfield Medical Center; at this point, we were just holding on to the hope offered to us by this faceless surgeon whom we had never met (and indeed would never meet) and about whom we knew nothing (other than the limited information discoverable through Google).

An hour later, as I was shuffling down the dreary hallway with Josh by my side in an effort to escape the claustrophobia of my room, someone came to tell me that the ambulance was on its way. Within minutes two EMTs were wheeling a gurney into my room, and I happily and very awkwardly climbed aboard. They fastened a belt around my middle; I was careful to hold the strap away from my distended stomach, to prevent compounding the pain and discomfort. They hoisted the gurney up and pushed me down the hallway, onto the elevator, and out the double doors into a waiting ambulance. I'd never been on a gurney or in an ambulance. Perhaps it was adrenaline pumping through my veins at finally getting out of that place, but I felt a bit of euphoria lying on that gurney, seeing the world from a completely new and exciting perspective.

During the summer before I started law school in 1999, I spent five weeks studying Spanish in Seville and then another five weeks backpacking alone through much of Europe. I was a little nervous about traveling alone—most people would be—but then add to that my visual limitations, and I was more than a little nervous. It was one of those things I had to do to prove to the world (but mostly to myself) that I could. I never booked accommodations in advance. I'd simply jump off the train in whatever new city, having just read the chapter on that city in my trusty guidebook, and look for a youth hostel using whatever map I could get my hands on. One warm summer night, with many more weeks to go in my travels, I was lying on a train platform, with my beloved purple backpack as a pillow, somewhere in the South of France, waiting for the next train that would take me to Rome. I was surrounded by a handful of other backpackers, yet entirely alone. I will never forget as I looked up at the starlit sky thinking that I had no idea where I would be sleeping the next night or the night after that or the night after that. And while there was a tinge of fear at the thought, I felt an overwhelming excitement for what lay ahead. There was a certain carefree joy in the not knowing, a freedom in not having to be anywhere or with anyone, in the promise of limitless possibilities. And then I felt an overwhelming sense of peace that chased away whatever trepidation I had, for I knew that everything would be okay, that I would find my way.

I felt that same way as I lay on the hoisted gurney, looking down at Josh as he walked beside me—yes, *down* at my six-foot-three Josh for a change. I had no idea what would happen the next day or the day after that or the day after that. In that moment, bizarrely, I was smiling with anticipation, excitement, and peace, off to the next adventure in my life. I bombarded the EMTs with questions, about where they came from, about whether they would turn on the sirens for me, about the most harrowing rescue they'd ever done.

As the ambulance raced onto the 10 freeway, heading west, toward the ocean, my eyes opened, and I began to wake from my nightmare and move from its darkness toward the light. And so began what I call the golden and magical part of my story of diagnosis.

18

A Love Story

The drive across Los Angeles was speedy, the freeways fortunately and bizarrely free of late-afternoon traffic. Within twenty-five minutes, I could smell the ocean and was staring up at the crystal-clear blue sky (another rarity for Los Angeles). The EMTs pushed me through the most beautiful hospital I had ever seen, brand spanking new, with wide and glistening hallways that seemed to go on forever, past orderlies, nurses, and doctors who smiled kindly at me, everything and everyone bathed in a soft golden light.

I expected to stop at a desk to satisfy some bureaucratic paperwork requirement, but no, the EMTs pushed me right into my own private room with a view of the Santa Monica Mountains and overlooking a quiet green courtyard (where my children would often play in the days to come), a flat-screen TV, real wood detailing, and three nurses clad in dark blue waiting to fuss over me. I had risen out of hospital hell and into hospital heaven.

The small army of nurses weighed me, changed my gown, started a new IV, drew blood, and got me a basin over which I hung my head as I begged for antinausea meds. Within half an hour of my arrival, Josh, who had driven there separately, walked through the door. And within twenty minutes of that, shortly after 5:00 P.M., my colorectal surgeon, Dr. D.C., with his chief resident, Dr. O., standing by his side—

both of them commanding, confident, and oh so reassuring in their crisp white coats—was telling us exactly what was going to happen. A gastroenterologist would go in that night at 8:30 to insert a stent to create an opening in my obstructed colon so that the waste trapped inside could flow out—an important step in preparing me for surgery to improve visibility and prevent postsurgical infection. If the gastro-enterologist could not place the stent, then Dr. D.C. and his team would be standing by to operate immediately. If the stent worked, then I would spend the next day and a half going to the bathroom so my bowels could be cleared, to be followed by surgery. As I listened and watched Dr. D.C. draw a picture of a colon on the white sheet on my bed, I thought, Now this is how medicine is supposed to be prac-ticed: dedicated surgeons immediately present and prepared to oper-ate late into the night to treat a patient they'd not known of four hours earlier.

I was consumed by the discomfort and nausea, trying hard not to throw up because I had been told that if I did, a tube would be stuck down my nose and into my stomach to suck my stomach's contents out, and I did not want that to happen. So all I could focus on were those parts of the conversation that dealt with the stent procedure and surgery; those were the only things that would give me physical relief.

But my husband was already thinking beyond that; he was thinking about the cancer itself and the future. I barely registered Josh's ques-tions to Dr. D.C. about whether he'd seen any evidence of metastases to other organs in the CT images we had brought from Garfield Medi-cal Center. No, Dr. D.C. said. They wouldn't know for sure until they went in, but he would guess I was probably Stage II or III. I was impa-tient at this line of conversation because all I wanted to do was get to the surgery, and that meant these men had to stop talking about cancer spread and staging and future treatments and if this and if that; none of that mattered right now; right now, I needed something to be done to relieve the nausea and pain.

Finally, Dr. D.C. left. Dr. O. presented me with some consent forms and told me about the risks of surgery, including something about the possibility that my bowels could not be put back in my body, in which case I would have an ostomy or colostomy or some other words that ended with "omy," and I nodded like I understood, even though I had no idea what he was talking about, and quickly signed the forms. Now I know what all of those words mean, but it was better that I didn't know back then. Soon, a cheerful Russian man in a green shirt came to wheel me to the procedure room. He was so happy, like everyone at that hospital, that I was convinced UCLA must pay its staff really well.

The stent was successfully placed that evening. When I woke from the hour-long procedure, I could feel the difference immediately. The release of pressure and pain was glorious. Sleep was elusive that night as I constantly and happily jumped out of bed and ran to the bathroom, dragging my IV pole behind me. Josh didn't sleep much that night, either, partly because of my frequent bathroom trips and partly because the recliner that would be his bed for the next few nights was not so comfortable. He told me how he would never have thought when we got married nearly six years earlier that he would be so happy to hear me pooping not five feet away from him. I had to laugh.

By morning, my stomach had returned to its usual size and softness, and I was feeling completely normal again, stretching and doing yoga poses, like I could run a mile or two or three—after all, up until I became symptomatic, a month earlier, I had probably been in the best shape of my life. Josh noted how my skin had its old glow again; only with the return of the old glow did we realize, though, how waxy and gray my face had grown over the last couple weeks, a visible yet unrecognized sign of the toxic waste trapped inside, poisoning my body. With the return of bowel function and the accompanying sense of normalcy, it was hard to imagine that there was a raging, murderous tumor inside me. But there was. That morning, without the official biopsy results from the colonoscopy back yet, Dr. D.C. came to tell us that my CEA was 53, whereas a normal CEA is less than 5. If there had been any part of us that had hoped I did not have cancer, that hope was completely erased by this news.

My surgery took place the next afternoon, on Wednesday, July 10. It was supposed to take two and a half hours but ended up taking four. Dr. D.C. would discover that my colon had grown to the size of a football and was already beginning to rupture, that in fact the unnaturally swollen part of my colon had pressed itself against my stomach in an attempt to keep itself intact; he marveled that my body had been able to adapt and hold my colon together, for a rupture would have been disastrous, throwing waste, colon, and cancer cells everywhere. The surgery was successful as my entire tumor (measuring 3.5 by 3.9 centimeters) and sixty-eight lymph nodes (twelve of which would prove to be cancerous), as well as the single drop metastasis on my peritoneum, were removed. Because the surgery was performed laparoscopically, recovery was a walk in the park, with bowel function returning thirty-six hours later, and minimal pain.

Once the surgery was over and the immediate emergency resolved, I had a lot of time to lie, sit, and sometimes walk aimlessly about, looking at and listening to the world around me but seeing and hearing nothing. I was too preoccupied with the business of beginning the lengthy process of absorbing and coming to grips with what had happened, was happening, and would likely happen to me.

On the day before surgery, July 9, when for the first time in days we felt "settled" and knew what the immediate next steps were, Josh had the energy and time to write an email with the subject line "Julie" to family and friends, some of whom we hadn't spoken to in years. The shock was immediate and total as family and friends called, texted, and emailed. I was morbidly curious to know how people reacted as they read the words, but I didn't ask. Did they collapse in a chair? Did they start crying? What did they think? Were they sad for me and Josh? Were they secretly relieved this hadn't happened to them? Were they afraid that it could?

Indeed, in addition to coming to terms with my own emotions, part of the acceptance process was absorbing and addressing the reactions of family and friends around me, sometimes allowing, but more often deflecting, their incredulity, horror, fears, sorrows, and hopes, sometimes permitting them to be my strength and comfort, and sometimes being theirs.

Of immediate concern to me was Josh. Rightly or wrongly, I've always felt that Josh is not as strong as I when it comes to handling life's challenges; I've had more practice than he; I'm a woman, and I firmly believe women are generally emotionally more capable and resilient. To be fair to Josh, though, I think my illness is much harder on him than it is on me, because he is the one who faces the prospect of going on without me to raise our children and pick up the pieces as I go forth into my next adventure beyond this life. It's always harder for the one left behind. But in those days after the surgery, I could not be his strength, certainly not nearly to the degree he needed. As he agonized and tried to find holes in the studies that offered the sobering statistics about Stage IV colon cancer, tried to spin the facts in the most favorable light possible (i.e., my relative youth, strength, access to the best medical care in the world, et cetera), he would drive me nuts. I would kick him out of my room to get breakfast at one of the many eateries in happening and trendy Santa Monica. I'd beg him to call his friends and family in New York and South Carolina, who were the foundation of his support system. I'd force him to go out for a beer with my brother or take our girls to the beach. I'd order him out in the evenings so he could go on solitary walks; exercise was important.

One night, he walked all the way to the pier, where he found an arcade with one of his favorite childhood games—Pac-Man. He played and he played until he had one quarter left. He made a deal then with himself, with God, with the forces of the universe in an attempt to peer into the future. If I break the record (a record set by someone else) with this last quarter, he told himself, then Julie will beat this cancer. He broke the record and came back to me giddy with excitement. So much for his steadfast belief in statistics . . .

The day after surgery—the day after we all knew I had Stage IV colon cancer—my sister (who had also made the trip to Los Angeles from New York for the family wedding and reunion) came to visit. She told me how she had not been able to sleep much of the night before, but then suddenly, as she was sitting in the dark, she was overcome by an absolute knowing that I would beat this cancer. She told me she just knew I would. I wished I had her blind faith. The next day she came to see me again, this time suddenly bursting into tears as she entered my room. This sister of mine who never cries hugged me and told me how I was the strong one, that I wasn't supposed to get sick, and how she had been trying to hold it together constantly around the girls and our parents, and now that they were all outside somewhere, she couldn't keep it pent up anymore. My sister was my daughters' surrogate mother during those early days. At my parents' house, while my mother made sure the girls were fed and bathed and as Josh slept in the hospital with me, Mia and Belle turned to my sister for comfort, cuddling against her every night because she was the closest thing to me that they had. My poor sister bore a heavy burden. I hugged her back, told her that indeed I was very strong, that I had always been and would always be.

Cousin N came to see me after work. She is notorious in our family for crying at anything and everything, but she'd been oddly stalwart since my diagnosis. I told her how I was astounded that she hadn't shed a single tear for me, secretly wondering if she didn't care as much as I thought she did. Oh, no, she said, just that day she'd cried a lot; she'd cried on the phone while talking to Cousin C, she'd cried at her desk afterward and to her co-workers, and she'd cried in her car, all the way to the hospital; but now she was all cried out; she was good for the time being. She flashed a smile that was a little too big, trying to hide the tears that glinted in the corners of her eyes. I think I loved Cousin N more than ever in that moment.

Even though I had frequent visitors, numerous phone calls, and much love, I spent many hours alone in my hospital room while everyone else was working or playing. Alone with my thoughts, my sadness, my fear, my shock. Fortunately, UCLA was my hospital heaven and angels abounded. I had and have stayed at other hospitals before and since, when I gave birth to my children and then after my HIPEC surgery, but there were no angels then, nothing particularly remarkable or memorable about the nurses who cared for me. There was something extraordinarily special about UCLA for me that I'd never known before and haven't known since. Perhaps another sign of God's hand in my life.

Karen, Noreen, Ray, Roxanne, Costa, Manuel, Ginger, Anita, Damian—names that mean nothing to you, but for me those names bring back memories of comfort and solace, hands, hugs, and words that consoled me in the darkest moments of my life. The people who are represented by those names were my true pillars of strength at a time when no one who loved me seemed to be able to bear the weight of my turbulent emotions, so for the most part I hid those emotions from the people I knew and loved, and instead unleashed them on these angels of mine. Their ability to listen, reassure, smile, and be optimistic in the face of all the horrors they saw every single day astounded and inspired me.

Costa clutched my hands one afternoon after she'd caught a glimpse of my girls leaving the room and prayed solemnly to God for me in a language I didn't understand. The fervor of her prayers brought tears to my eyes. Then she went about changing my sheets.

Karen, the twenty-six-year-old Chinese American woman—a girl, really—who reminded me so of my good friend V, accompanied me on many a walk around the floor, telling me about how when she saw my name, she had been taken aback because Yip had also been the name of her mother, who died at age thirty-eight of colon cancer when Karen was only two years old, leaving behind her overwhelmed father and three grieving older siblings. I could feel that Karen took comfort in me as much as I took comfort in her. I could feel that hand of God again when I looked into her strangely familiar face.

Then there was the man whose name I never knew, the one who didn't speak a word of English, whom I might have mistaken for a youthful gangster in any other setting in light of the way his dark brown hair was slicked back into a ponytail at the nape of his neck and the way the rippling muscles in his forearms bespoke an easy violence if he so chose. He silently cleaned me one night after I'd had a humiliating accident. The gentleness of his touch, and the absence of disgust and judgment, which I found shocking and so humbling, destroyed all my unkind preconceived notions of who he was. I doubted that I could do for a stranger what he was doing for me, but I wanted to after being in his presence. I witnessed through him the extent and power of compassion, the love that one human being can express to another through action alone, not because they know one another but because they are simply members of the same human race.

And then there was David, my colorectal surgeon, whose nimble hands removed sixty-eight lymph nodes, an extraordinary number that was a testament to his exceptional skill and tenacity. I've yet to meet anyone who has had sixty-eight lymph nodes removed laparoscopically. As I've often been told, the best odds for survival begin with a skilled surgeon, and I had the best surgeon I could possibly have had. He is my age, and he and his wife are Chinese American, and have two children, too, who are about the same ages as Mia and Belle. David spent hours answering our questions, going over the incomprehensible color photos from the surgery with Josh and me, reviewing the results of the pathology and scan reports, punching holes in the troubling studies, and then telling Josh not to "perseverate," filling my head with stories of patients who had overcome against all odds.

I'm sure David felt sorry for us—a young family much like his own coming out to Los Angeles for vacation and then being blindsided by an advanced cancer diagnosis. I would have felt sorry for me, too. But even so, he did more than a typical compassionate doctor would have done. He befriended us (or as much as he could, given the doctor-patient dynamics of our relationship). When he heard that we were looking for a short-term rental nearby so I could recuperate, he offered us an unused part of his house. We didn't think he was actually serious, so we just ignored the offer.

At the end of our monthlong stay in L.A., on the evening before we were to fly back to New York, he invited us to his rambling house perched on the side of a canyon, for a playdate with the kids and dinner. It was then that we realized he'd actually been sincere in his offer of a place to stay. Our kids played with ladybugs and puzzles that focused on the different parts of the human body while the adults drank and ate cheese, mussels, pasta, and ice cream. It was a lovely evening, reinforcing my belief that under different circumstances, we would have been true friends. At the end of the evening, as we said our goodbyes, I stood there facing an uncertain and terrifying future and facing David, this man who had seen and removed the raging, murderous tumor in me. I tried to find the words to express my gratitude. How do you say thank you to the person who has seen your insides and saved your life? Is it even possible? No words came. I made a helpless gesture with my hand that was supposed to mean "thank you," and then I broke down in tears. We hugged, and he cried, too. And then he looked at me and told me, "You're going to be fine, just fine."

My Chinese last name means leaf. The Chinese love their idiomatic sayings, where four syllables can carry deep and profound meaning.

There is one in particular that I associate with my time in Los Angeles, both while at UCLA and in the weeks after, and that is "A fallen leaf always returns to its roots." I was undeniably a fallen leaf then, and I had returned to the place where I grew up, where so much of my family and so many friends remain, and where new friends gathered, where they encircled me, Josh, and our girls in love and protection, where I started the process of rebirth into a new life. My parents would go back and forth between their home and the hospital and then later the rental, toting food and our laundered clothes, chargers, toiletries, and anything else we needed. Cousin N and her husband offered a bed and shower at her nearby apartment so Josh could freshen up in a place more comfortable than my hospital bathroom.

Family and friends offered playdates and other fun and distracting activities for my girls. Third Aunt and Uncle came to visit in the hospital, donning hazard masks and gowns before they entered my room (for this was when I was still being tested for *C. difficile,* and precautions had to be taken to prevent the spread of any bacteria). Fifth Aunt and Uncle made the long drive after work from the east side to visit me. Other aunts and uncles whom I hadn't spoken to in years showed up to tell me they loved me. Yes, Chinese people telling me they loved me; that was nearly as shocking as being told I had cancer. In a true gesture of love, they cooked me feast after feast to try to fatten me up. My family and friends threw a big party to celebrate Belle's second birthday and as a celebration of life for me, to which family and friends from different walks of my life came, some of them traveling thousands of miles to be there.

While in some respects the story of my diagnosis was a nightmare, I think it is ultimately a story of love between me and all those who came to support me. In my moments of elusive faith, I believed the hand of God had brought me to Los Angeles then so that I could know that kind of magical and singular love, a love that I had never experienced before and, I daresay, that even many of those who have lived many more years than I have never experienced and will never experience. Sadly, it's the type of love that is shown only when life is threatened, when for a few minutes, hours, days, or weeks, everyone agrees on and understands what really matters. And yet, as transient as that love can be, its magic, intensity, and power can sustain the most cynical among us, as long as we allow ourselves to linger in the glow of its memory. This disease may bring me to the final days of my life on this earth, but the story of how cancer came into my life reminds me every day that while it has taken from me the innocence and happiness of my old life, it has also given me the gift of human love, which has now become part of my soul and which I will take with me forever.

19

Fate and Fortune

When I learned that my parents and grandparents tried to kill me, it didn't just make me feel a thousand different volatile emotions; it also made me think those grand thoughts and pose those mind-numbing questions that theologians and philosophers have been pondering and raising for millennia. But fortunately, unlike the raw emotions running through my body, these thoughts and questions were, for the most part, comfortingly familiar and calming in their intellectual nature, as I'd been pondering and raising the same ones in some form or fashion since I was a little girl.

From the moment I was capable of somewhat advanced thinking and realized that I was different, and not necessarily in a good way, I began compiling a list of questions that grew in length and sophistication as I grew, a list of questions for the Buddhist gods and local Chinese saints I had known in my childhood, my ancestors who might as well have been gods, the Christian God that all Americans believed in it seemed, at least based on what the television was telling me, and any other Being who might be out there. I must have been six or seven when I began the list. Through the years, I would stare up at the ceiling on sleepless, frustrated nights and present my list.

Buddha, Goddess of the Sea, Great-Great-Grandfather, God, All Powerful and Knowing Being, if any of you has the time to listen to

me, can you please answer some questions for me? I need to understand.

Why was I born blind?

Why couldn't I have been born in this country, where the doctors
could have fixed me with a snap of their fingers?

Why didn't we make it to America sooner, because sooner would
have meant more vision?

Of all the bodies in this world I could have been born into, why this
body with the fucked-up eyes?

Is there a reason, a greater purpose, for me being born into this
body, in a poor country, and at a turbulent time? Because, you know, if
there were, that would make my fucked-up vision and the hurt so
much easier to deal with.

What is that greater purpose?

And what is to come next in my life? What lies in my future? What
am I supposed to do?

After my mother told me what she'd done, I reasked all those questions and added another question to the top of the list:

Why did I live when I could have so easily died?

After each question, I would pause, listening carefully for an answer and looking for a sign that might be an answer. No answers ever
came, not when I was eight, not when I was eighteen, and not when I
was twenty-eight. Without any answers, the questions became inner
musings, evolving over the years into metaphysical discussions that
took place entirely inside my head. Instead of answers, they produced
more questions.

Well, maybe it was all an accident. Maybe there's no reason for any
of it and I should be happy and grateful that things just happened to
work out the way they did.

But how can all of this, this whole world, our convoluted, complicated lives, be a gigantic accident? How can people suffer from dis-
abling diseases and die for no reason? How can suffering and death be
matters of sheer bad luck?

No, there must be a point to it all. There must be a plan for me, for
everyone, put in motion by a god or the gods, our ancestors, the universe, Someone or Something. And maybe in the end, all we can do is

live and make the best choices we can, and everything will just work out . . .

But that's unacceptable! Am I, are we all, supposed to just flail around hoping that there's some plan out there and that no matter what we do, it'll all be okay in the end? I mean, how do I know what choices are best? How do I know what the plan is? And if there really is a plan and a reason for every horrible thing that happens to us in this world and everything has been predetermined, what is the point of doing anything at all, because self-will and free choice would be utterly meaningless. Why should we do anything to make the horrible things not so horrible?

I started looking elsewhere for my answers. I must have been about twelve when we got a free copy of one of the Mysteries of the Unknown books when my brother or sister subscribed to *Time* magazine. Mysteries was a series that explored the strange and the unexplained— UFOs, hauntings, witchcraft—but the book we got was about psychic powers. Pages were devoted to the art of palm reading, depicting differently shaped palms with various line patterns. I was captivated and comforted by the idea that a person's character and future could be discerned from the lines on his hand, because that would mean that there is a set plan and we don't have to flounder about in this universe with its frighteningly infinite possibilities. I watched with fascination when self-proclaimed psychics appeared on *Donahue, Geraldo, The Sally Jessy Raphael Show,* and *Larry King Live,* people who could see the future through reading palms, tarot cards, or tea leaves, read the auras of the living, or talk to the prescient spirits of the dead. Now, these were people who might be able to answer all my questions or connect me to the Beings who could.

Even though I knew that there were many frauds out there who fueled the skeptics' arguments, believing that there were true clairvoyants was not a stretch for me since I came from a family culture that embraced a bit of Buddhism and lots of popular religion, which itself consisted of healthy doses of ancestor worship and old-world superstitions. When I was growing up in Southern California, the world of fortune-tellers, of spirits and ghosts, of all those invisible things that move in some supernatural dimension was real, part of my experience through the stories my mother told of the old country and through the rituals of our everyday lives. Ghosts had been known to roam our house in Tam Ky, washing dishes and cleaning floors in the dead of night. The woman who sold tobacco on the streets of Tam Ky (the one married to the Da Nang herbalist) and the spirit of her deceased grandfather, who returned to this world by occupying the body of a teenage boy to give aid to the living, were celebrated characters in my family lore. After all, it was the Grandfather Spirit who had told us that we had to leave Vietnam when we did. "After your boat leaves, no more boats will leave from here. If you miss this boat, you will have lost your chance for a long time, maybe forever," he warned my paternal grandmother as his host's body shook with unearthly tremors. My mother's parents and all her siblings were supposed to depart on the next boat, due to depart only several weeks after ours, but that boat never left. My maternal grandmother asked the Grandfather Spirit then when they would be able to get out. "Ten years" was his response. I met my mother's parents and all her siblings at Los Angeles International Airport exactly ten years later.

My family was not so blessed as to have the spirits of our benevolent ancestors come back to us in human form, but we still sought their help. Our family rituals included frequent offerings and prayers to our ancestors, long-deceased great-grandparents and great-great-grandparents, who in death became godlike in their omniscience and omnipotence. On the first and fifteenth day of every lunar month, Chinese New Year, and Death Day, the day on which the dead are remembered, my mother would set up in the front doorway of our house a candlelit table full of fruits, fish, chicken, pork, rice, tea, and wine. Bundles of incense burned on the table, the fragrant wisps of smoke inviting the Buddhist gods and our ancestors' spirits to come feast and listen to our prayers. We also tried to fulfill our ancestors' material desires for riches they did not have on earth. On the death anniversaries of those ancestors who had been closest to us—my great-grandmother and later my grandmother—and on Death Day, we would throw into a flame-spewing metal drum stacks of shiny, gold-colored paper—money in the afterlife—along with red mansions, blue Mercedes, robust-looking servants, and tailored clothes, all made of paper. Within seconds, the flames transformed our offerings into black ash, releasing clouds of dark smoke that lifted toward the heavens, carrying the riches to our beloved.

"Ask for whatever you want, and if you are respectful and honor the gods and our ancestors, they will listen to you," my mother taught me. Following her lead, I would stand behind the offering table, holding one or three or five sticks of smoking incense (never an even number, for that was bad luck), close my eyes tight, thank the gods and my ancestors for the goodness they had shown us, and then ask them for things big and small—health for everyone in my family, lots of money next Chinese New Year, straight A's on the next report card, normal vision . . . and most of the time, I got what I asked for.

The gods and our ancestors were constants in our home. We felt and were comforted by the eyes of the Buddha statues and of our ancestors, whose images were memorialized forever in dusty, framed black-and-white photos, some of which had been brought over from the old country. They followed us from their perches atop the family altar, situated on the fireplace mantel or a mounted platform, where red, pointy bulbs, which were supposed to imitate real candles, always shone and incense always burned, browning the ceiling above. After my grandmother died, we could feel her in every creak of the house in the night, every movement of a door not caused by a human touch, every flickering of a light. "There goes Grandma," we would say. For six months after my grandmother died, as her spirit made its gradual way to the next world and before she found her place on the family altar, we left an empty seat at the dinner table so she could eat with us. In front of the seemingly vacant chair would be a bowl full of rice, with a pair of chopsticks standing straight up in the middle of the rounded mound of white. When the grief was so fresh right after her death, we remembered not to sit in her seat, but as the months passed and as the other world called to her more and more, we began to forget and someone would sit in her chair at dinner, I or Lyna or Mau or one of the cousins. "Don't sit on Grandma!" someone would yell, and the offender would guiltily jump out of her seat.

Even though I felt we tried so hard to make our ancestors happy and to speak to them so that they would hear us, they never seemed to speak to us or guide us in the way I wanted, in the way the Grandfather Spirit had guided my grandmother and mother years ago. Where was his equivalent for me? I needed my questions answered, too.

My confusion and frustrations with the gods, saints, and spirits of my childhood only grew with age, and especially after I left home for college. Still, in the beginning of my college years, I missed them, those unseen and unresponsive Beings with whom I had lived for seventeen years. I felt at times bereft in my new Waspy environment, three thousand miles away from ever-warm Southern California, longing for the comforts of home, which included the rituals of offering and prayer I had always known and taken for granted. In that idyllic college town in the mountains of western Massachusetts—where a Congregational church housed in a two-hundred-year-old white colonial building and an Episcopal church housed in an even older Gothic edifice sat in the middle of campus against the spectacular reds, oranges, and yellows of my first fall foliage and then the blinding white of my first New England snow—I felt a little out of place. There was not one pair of chopsticks or a single Buddha statue to be found, except, in the case of the Buddha statue, maybe buried in a photo in one of the books stored in the East Asian section of the 10-million-volume college library.

At first, I tried to perform the rituals of home in my dorm room, but on a much more modest and inconspicuous scale. I placed a little can filled with grains of uncooked rice on my windowsill, overlooking a brick building with ivy climbing up its walls. The can was positioned right next to a Gregorian-lunar desk calendar that reminded me in Chinese characters which were the days for me to speak to the gods and my ancestors. And on those days, when my roommate wasn't around, I went through the motions of lighting one or three or five sticks of incense and praying and then standing the incense in the can of rice, just like we did at home. I realized then that my mother had never taught me how to carry on the rituals myself, to establish the lines of communication without her there. What was I supposed to say to call the Beings to me? How was I supposed to address them? I felt like a fraud, playing pathetically at being a Buddhist, ancestor worshipper, practitioner of popular religion, and whatever else I was supposed to be.

I had never thought to ask my mother about the philosophy behind all this, why we bothered to do all this offering and praying, where the source of her faith in these invisible gods and spirits lay—probably because I had a feeling she didn't know the answers to those questions herself. She didn't know the teachings of the Buddha any more than I did. She performed the rituals because she had seen her mother do it, and her mother had seen *her* mother do the same; these were unquestioned family traditions that had been passed from one generation to the next in the old country, where every family did the same. My following of those same traditions seemed empty, even on this modest scale, on this liberal arts college campus that had felt at first so alien but was growing more familiar every day, where I was being encouraged to think, to question, and if I was so moved, to reject. I stopped performing my prayer rituals regularly after the first semester, although I did not stop presenting my list of unanswered questions to any Being that might be listening.

Armed with that new sense of freedom and possibility that comes with college life, not to mention hard-earned work-study money and a credit card, I began unconsciously searching for my Grandfather Spirit equivalent one autumn night during my sophomore year. Bored in a college town with not much to do on a Saturday night except drink, my friend Sue and I fell victim to the persuasive power of years of late-night commercials—we called the Psychic Hotline. "Come on, Sue. It'll be fun," I urged my wary friend. Sue and I both knew there was an incredibly high likelihood that it would be bogus, although I was secretly hoping against reason that we might actually encounter the real thing, and I guess so was Sue, since she agreed.

I dialed the 976 number, punching the little white buttons of my bright blue plastic phone, which looked more like a toy with which my baby cousins might play than something that could serve as a bridge to the psychic forces of the universe. A machine asked me to punch in my credit card number. I punched. Then a click.

"Thank you for calling the Psychic Hotline, where all the secrets of your future will be revealed," said the guy on the other end of the line. He sounded like he was either half asleep or stoned out of his mind. I could tell then that this was not going to go well. When he told me that based on my aura I was going to be pregnant within the year, if I wasn't already, I rolled my eyes and wordlessly handed the phone over to Sue. She hung up on the guy after he told her she had a tilted uterus, which was why she suffered severe cramps every month. Today we still laugh and cringe at that idiotic waste of twenty dollars.

Still, the Psychic Hotline experience did not deter us. During spring break of that year, which we spent in L.A., Sue and I were lured into a tiny store on Melrose Avenue, its window adorned with the pink flashing neon message PALM READING $5. The gypsy woman inside—at least that was how she was dressed—with the Transylvanian accent foretold over a crystal ball that I would find my true love in six months (which I did not) and that Sue would find much professional success in some way that the woman could not specify. Sue stopped seeing alleged psychics with me after that experience, and I went on alone in my search.

After the Psychic Hotline and the Melrose Avenue palm reader was the Tibetan Buddhist palm-reading monk, whom I encountered during my junior year abroad in western China; he declared that I was incredibly intelligent. After him came the palm-reading fisherman I found along the Yangzi River, who predicted that I would have a long, successful life. Next was the Chinese astrologer of Taipei, who said nothing memorable. Then there was the Turkish tea-leaves reader of Sierra Madre, California, who said I would have a great time on my next vacation. And of course, there was Clairvoyant Mark of New York City, the aura and palm reader at the drunken company holiday party at the Rainbow Room, who also said I was smart.

Yet among this parade of unremarkable, if not altogether bad, readings and observations, there was one woman who was quite unforgettable, not because she could predict my future but because she could see into my past.

She was a palm reader. I met her five years before my mother told me about what she and the rest of them had tried to do to me. After I learned that, this woman's words would come back to me with greater impact; it was almost like she knew before I knew.

We had met in her high-rise apartment on the east side of midtown Manhattan. Daylight streamed into the giant windows that overlooked Third Avenue. The apartment was not what I had come to expect.

There were no candles, no chairs or sofas covered in red velour, no plastic beads hanging in the doorway between her living room and her inner sanctum, no gold-tasseled tablecloths and cushions, no crystal ball. Instead, the apartment was decorated in muted tans and browns with carefully coordinated splashes of color in the throw pillows on the sofa and in the lush rugs. I wouldn't have minded living in such a space. The woman herself was an extension of the apartment. Dressed in cream-colored pants and a white sweater with a clean, barely made-up face, this middle-aged woman did not look to me like someone able to see what the rest of us could not.

I had really come to her apartment to hire her services for a big bash my roommates and I were throwing that coming weekend. As part of our commitment to live fully our never-again-to-be-experienced carefree postcollege years in New York City, we had decided to invite everyone we could think of to invade our seven-hundred-square-foot, three-bedroom apartment on the Upper East Side for an unforgettable party. A fortune-teller would help to make it unforgettable, I had suggested. The roommates enthusiastically embraced my suggestion, so I had been assigned the task of finding the fortune-teller. In the end, I liked the price this woman had given me over the phone. I had come to her apartment to meet her face-to-face and to make sure that she was legitimate, or at least that she wasn't going to murder us all. And just maybe, I thought, I would allow myself to be the guinea pig to see if she was—on the off chance—the real thing.

After we finished discussing the logistics for the party, she agreed to read my palm for twenty-five dollars for one half hour—a reasonable price—and without that icky eagerness that would have hinted at a woman desperate for business. I liked that. I was cautiously optimistic.

We sat across from one another at a little smoky glass table. She flipped on the lamp next to us, its light bright enough to uncover the darkest mysteries, I thought. Then she slipped her frameless reading glasses on her nose, snapping shut their case with a quick *thwack*. She held out her hands toward me.

"Now I have to see both your palms," she said.

I met her halfway, extending my arms so that my palms rested between us, their countless lines staring up at both of us.

"For a woman, her right palm tells the truth about her life as she now lives it, while her left palm reveals clues into what her life might have been in her alternate fate."

Well, that was new to me, and a fascinating notion, if true.

Her cool hands were white against mine, her light green veins pronounced, her fingernails neat ovals with clear polish. She grazed the lines of one palm with her fingertips and then bent my fingers on both hands back farther than I thought they could go, lowering her head another couple inches to scrutinize the tiniest lines. Then after what seemed like endless minutes of silence, interrupted only by the sound of my own breathing, she looked up at me.

"Well, your palms are very interesting," she said quite deliberately.

Yep, just stalling to give yourself more time to make up something grand, I'll bet. I hope at least you come up with something a little more original or else I'm really going to feel like a moron (yet again) for wasting money.

"There is a big difference between your right and left palms, a very dramatic difference," she continued. "In the right one, I see a good long life. You see how your life line goes all the way down here and how deep it is?" She traced the line with her right index finger.

Sure, I guess so.

Not waiting for a response, she went on. "But then look at the life line on your left palm. It's short, and there are so many lines cutting into it. This palm tells me that in your alternate life, you would have suffered much illness, frustration, and unhappiness, and early death."

Okay, now that's original.

She looked up again. "There must have been a profound change in your life. Something happened that truly altered the course your life would have taken," she said, clearly intrigued by the story my palms were telling her.

I had made it a policy to not help these fortune-tellers, to give them minimal information about myself, but sometimes they did need something a little bit more specific and concrete to guide them along.

"Well, I left home a few years ago and decided to live far away from my family," I offered. That was nice and vague but still somewhat informative.

She gave her head a quick shake. "No, no. That might be part of it, but it's not that. There's something else, something that happened when you were little." The woman seemed genuinely puzzled and bothered. I decided to take some pity on her, to tell her part of what had instantly come to my mind when she mentioned illness and frustration.

"Well, I was born in Vietnam and came here when I was almost four years old. That certainly changed my life very dramatically."

She was looking at me again, peering intently over the top of her glasses in a way that made me just a little uneasy. "Yes, that makes more sense. But I think there's more to it . . . It has to do with your eyes, doesn't it?" Her voice trailed off, as if she were musing to herself and not aloud to me.

Some people think that I just have thick glasses. Most of the time I can move around with my bad vision pretty well, almost like a normally sighted person. Others, the people who are a little more observant, will notice the never-ending quivering of my pupils and will guess that there's something more going on than the typical eye afflictions. In any case, almost no one ever has the nerve to mention it to me or, worse yet, ask me directly about it, for fear of offending me. So I was a little startled by this woman's bluntness. I liked it, though; it was refreshing. And for her to connect my eye problem with what she was seeing in my palms, well, that was kind of brilliant, I had to admit. I answered her question.

"I couldn't see when I was born in Vietnam, and I didn't get surgery to fix the problem until I came to America—as much as they could fix at that point, because it was pretty late in the game. I imagine my life would have been very different had I not made it to this country," I explained.

"Well then, you're one lucky girl," the palm reader stated. She said it with the confidence of a well-accepted fact, as simple as two plus two equals four.

"I suppose so. I've not always thought of myself that way, to be honest. Sometimes it's hard to deal with, not being able to see like the rest of the world, and all you can focus on is everything that you can't do. It really sucks, you know." To my great surprise, I found myself choking up as I talked. I had to stop before it became obvious to this total stranger. Sometimes this happened, as if all the self-indulgent emotions I bottled up threatened to come to the surface and expose me.

Still, it's funny how you can feel comfortable enough to tell a perfect stranger deeply personal things. Sometimes you just need someone to listen to you. Knowing that I would never see her one-on-one again and that she had no preconceived notions about me just made it easier somehow.

She was patient and kind. "What your palms are telling me, what they're telling you if you knew how to read them, is that you should focus on how far you've come from where you began in your life. Be happy about that. Something that some people don't realize is that the lines on a person's palm can change and do change all the time. Your future is not set in stone. In the beginning, there are many things that we have no control over—where we are born, who our parents are, how we come into this world with something wrong with our eyes or maybe our ears or our legs, whatever it is—but from there it's up to us to decide what we do with what we've been given. We make our own choices."

I have often imagined what my life could have been in some alternate universe where different choices, in which I had no say, were made at critical moments that might or might not have seemed so critical at the time, choices in moments that forever defined the course of my life. What if my mother had never taken those green pills she suspects caused my blindness? What if our boat had planned to leave Vietnam only weeks later, at the same time my mother's parents were supposed to leave? What if my mother had decided not to marry my father? What if the herbalist had been willing to do the unthinkable? There are infinite possibilities that make up that alternate universe. But there were only two, and then later three, basic scenarios that haunted my imagination most.

In Scenario One, I am born normal, or I am born in the United States, or come over within the first six months of my life so my eyes are fixed completely by the doctors here, who seem like miracle workers to most people in the world. I can see perfectly. I can do anything

and everything—play tennis, drive a car, climb mountains. I am beautiful and popular because I'm not a freak with my Coke-bottle glasses,
my giant large-print books, and my many magnifying glasses. I grow
up as a normal kid. Scenario One made me hurt and sad for everything
that could have been. It was what I longed for when I was angry, frustrated, and self-pitying. My mother shared my longing for this perfect
world. I know, because when my GPA fell short of a 4.0 or when she
saw me struggling down a set of stairs, she would say, unable to sup-
press the impulse, "It's so too bad. Imagine what more you could have
done if you could see normally. If only the doctors had been able to fix
it completely . . ." I could say nothing in response because she was
right. I could imagine.

In Scenario Two, I am alone, trapped behind the blinding whiteness
of cataracts. We never make it out of Vietnam. I am always wearing
old, faded clothes with holes my mother has patched. They hang on
my thin, malnourished body. I cling to my mother because I have no
white cane. I never leave the house in Tam Ky because my family is
afraid that I will get run over by a car. I never go to school because no
one teaches the blind in Vietnam. Scenario Two humbled me in gratitude. It was what I envisioned when I tried to overcome the anger,
frustration, and self-pity. My mother never spoke of this scenario. She
didn't have to, because I know its very real possibility underlay her
desperate desire to leave Vietnam, more so than even the desperate
desire for economic and political freedom. "We left Vietnam because
we wanted your eyes to be fixed," she would say.

And then, five years after I encountered this palm reader, when my
mother told me what she did, I imagined Scenario Three: I am dead at
age two months. Scenario Three makes me hurt, sad, and humbled. It
always rests within my soul. Except for when my mother revealed the
truth to me, no one ever talks about this scenario, perhaps because at
one point it had nearly been a foregone conclusion.

After my encounter with the palm reader, in the midst of living life,
of studying and working and going on vacations, of having dinner
with friends, of gossiping away on the phone with my cousins about
the ordinary and extraordinary events of our lives, of working out at
the gym and kayaking in the Antarctic, of falling in love and getting

married, the palm reader's words finally began to seep into my stubborn brain and heart. I know this because somewhere along the way, I stopped asking the gods my list of questions with the same old frequency. Maybe my alternate universe was really not the beautiful and perfect but wistful dream of Scenario One, the loss of which I had often mourned. Rather, perhaps it was the more probable tragic fates of Scenarios Two and Three, which I had managed to escape somehow. "Illness," "frustration," "unhappiness," and "early death" the palm reader had said of my alternate universe. "Lucky" she had said of my fate up to that point. We decide for ourselves how to deal with what we have been given; it's our choice, she had said. For so long, I had been overly concerned with figuring out the purpose and reason for the oh-so-terrible circumstances of my birth, the universe's plan for me, and what was going to come next, so much that I had discounted the importance of free choice.

The palm reader was trying to let me know that, if I would only listen and look, my palms were telling me the story of my life, of how far I had come from where I began, a place fraught with unfortunate circumstances beyond my control, but where and how far I had traveled in my life, while somewhat determined by historic and familial forces also beyond my control, was largely determined by me. The future would not seem so overwhelming with its infinite possibilities if I looked at my palms for the story of my past, to find comfort in the good choices made and the hard lessons learned. Could it be that after years of unsuccessfully looking without and to the invisible Beings of the heavens for the answers to my questions, I could actually find them by looking down at my own palms, within myself, and to my own past?

Little did I then know of the further choices I would have to make, and of the even harder lessons I would learn.

20

Numbers, a Reassessment

Somewhere, the outcome of all of this is known—everything from the largest to the smallest, including our little lives. Numbers are just the way we try to calculate the future.

At the beginning of this cancer detour, when faced with the sobering statistics, for my own self-preservation I intuitively shunned the numbers, insisting to myself and Josh as well that I am someone who has always defied the odds and that this would be no different. I knew I wasn't a number.

Since then, I've portrayed Josh as the steadfast adherent to science, studies, and statistics on one side and me as the staunch believer in self, faith, and all that is unquantifiable on the other. As another autumn comes on and I am still alive, sixteen months after my diagnosis, I have come to realize that those two sides, theoretically representing two opposing perspectives, are not so opposite or cut and dried, that indeed numbers don't just mean squat, that they are informative and valuable. But they must be understood within a nuanced context that overly simplistic statements like "You are not a number" don't even begin to capture.

A Tuesday in October 2014 was our seventh wedding anniversary, and it seems only fitting that I should write something to honor our marriage. I am happy to report that the state of our union is strong and good, that we fight less, communicate better, and if possible love each other more than we did a year ago, and certainly about a thousand times more than we did the day we married. It might sound like a funny subject for a love note, but I wanted to mark this anniversary by resolving our longstanding disagreement over the virtues and faults of statistics.

The night before my diagnostic laparoscopy, as I agonized over what tomorrow would bring and my future, remembering as always the stated odds of me beating Stage IV colon cancer, and with the thought of our wedding anniversary still at the forefront of my mind, I asked Josh, "What were the odds of us getting married when we were born?"

He posited, "Zero."

Because Josh and I come from such different worlds, separated not just by physical distance, but also by culture, war, politics, education, and even my blindness, I've often marveled at how we managed to find one another and fall in love. I've wondered what we were each doing at the various defining moments of our respective lives apart.

While he was born into the relative comfort and luxury of Greenville, South Carolina, into an insular and genteel world of southern charm and propriety, my ten-month-old self was living on the other side of the earth in a subtropical world of monsoons and rice paddies, in the throes of extreme poverty and ethnic and economic persecution as the Communists sought retribution against those who had defied them during the war. Government thugs were on the brink of occupying my family's home and confiscating all our personal property to contribute to the collective that stood at the core of the socialist ideal. While Josh's grandmother was bragging about her three-year-old grandson's uncanny ability to read at such a young age, I had not yet seen a written word and had instead just immigrated to the United States, a nearly yearlong journey that began one dark night as we all boarded trucks bound for the harbor where an unseaworthy fishing boat awaited its three hundred passengers.

On the evening my mother removed the bandages from my eyes after my first surgery and at age four I saw for the first time a relatively unclouded world, Josh must have already been fast and cozily asleep in his bed three thousand miles away, so obviously full of a unique intelligence and potential that was presumed to be completely lacking in me. While I skipped a day of school to celebrate Chinese New Year in January or February of each year, to collect red envelopes filled with money, listen to firecrackers go *pop pop pop* at least three hundred times, and make our annual trip to a Buddhist temple to pray, Josh had a normal day at his parochial school, where I assume he went to chapel and then moved quickly through the material that had been assigned for that day, much more quickly than how I progressed at my poorly ranked public school in Los Angeles. While he ate turkey on Thanksgiving and opened presents on Christmas Day, I watched TV or read a book or played with my cousins, like it was any other day we had off from school. When I ponder the disparate worlds from which Josh and I hailed, I do believe he is right, that the odds thirty-eight years ago of us ever getting married were pretty close to 0 percent, if not actually 0 percent.

But yet, we did meet and marry. In this chaotic universe of so many people and innumerable paths crossing randomly for brief moments of time, our life threads touched and fused together. If the odds of us meeting and getting married were 0 percent when we were babies, as Josh and I both believe, then how did we in fact meet and get married? How can that impossible occurrence be reconciled with the numbers? Is it as simple as that our union is an example of how numbers mean squat, that indeed our union is proof positive of the worthlessness of statistics? If I ever thought that to be true, I don't anymore.

If I didn't believe in the numbers that tell me I will likely not die when I walk out the door or board a plane, if I didn't believe in the numbers that tell me my children will likely not be shot by some madman invading their school, then I would never leave our home, and would certainly never let my children leave, either. We go to bed every night expecting the sun to rise in the morning because based on the rules of probability, this is what will happen. We save for our children's college educations and our own retirements because based on the odds, we expect our children to grow up healthy and go to college, and yes, we expect ourselves to age and enjoy retirement. Everything we do in our lives, we do based on the likelihood of something happening; it's called planning.

While those of us who have advanced cancer would like to ignore the statistics that pertain to whether we will live or die from our disease and to say that numbers mean squat, it would be hypocritical to do so, because even as we live with our disease, we must in fact continue to *live*, and with living comes the need to plan. I must still believe in the numbers; otherwise, I wouldn't—couldn't—do anything; I wouldn't cross the street; I wouldn't agree to undergo exhausting treatments that statistically have proven to be at least somewhat effective; I wouldn't plan birthday parties or vacations. I do all these things because despite the improbability of my getting sick in the first place, I still expect the earth to rotate, the universe to operate based on certain rules, and the outcomes that the statistics predict to actually happen. I cannot pick and choose which numbers to live by because I don't like the predicted outcome.

But odds are not prophecy, and what is expected to happen sometimes doesn't happen. Plans fall apart. Children grow up and show no interest in college despite their parents' best efforts. Adults die, leaving their retirement funds untapped. Madmen invade schools and slaughter the innocent. People with Stage I cancer years later experience a recurrence and die from metastatic cancer, even though the odds were heavily in their favor at diagnosis, and people with Stage IV cancer somehow live far longer than anyone would have expected. And maybe someday the earth will be struck by a giant asteroid that will obliterate all life as we know it. And when those unlikely events happen, the probability of their occurrence becomes 100 percent.

Josh has a not-quite-immobilizing fear of flying. Even so, he has a morbid fascination with air disasters, and so he (and therefore I) have watched endless hours of air disaster shows on National Geographic and the Smithsonian Channel, shows with C-class actors reenacting the last harrowing minutes of a commercial airliner's flight before it crashes into the side of a mountain, a quiet neighborhood, or the ocean, and the investigative efforts to uncover what went wrong. Sometimes there are happy endings, in which by some miracle the pilots manage to save passengers and crew. But that rarely happens.

Everyone knows that flying is statistically significantly safer than driving, that given the number of people who fly around the world and the few accidents there are, flying is the safest form of travel. Of course, as Josh and I watch an episode, we both are thinking that my odds of beating Stage IV colon cancer are much better than the odds of those people on that flight living more than two minutes; anything is better than a 0 percent likelihood of survival, the odds for those doomed people. I've asked Josh why, if he's afraid of flying, he likes to watch these shows. He tells me because they perversely make him feel better, reinforcing to him how many things must happen for an air disaster to occur, that in essence it's the coalescing of a multitude of random and unlikely occurrences—the perfect storm.

Josh's current obsession is with Air France Flight 447, a flight from Rio to Paris that crashed in the Atlantic Ocean in June 2009, killing all 228 people onboard. (He has forced me to watch the episode at least twenty times by now—the things you do for those you love . . .) A storm caused ice crystals to form in the plane's pitot tubes, which in turn caused a temporary and what would ordinarily be a minor inconsistency and malfunction in the plane's airspeed measurements, which in turn caused the autopilot to disconnect, which in turn forced two young and inexperienced copilots to take control of the plane. It just so happened that after a night of partying in Rio with his girlfriend and on little sleep, the seasoned captain had chosen only moments earlier to go for his scheduled and authorized nap. The two copilots panicked in response to the erroneous readings of slowed airspeed, instinctively pushing the airplane's nose up (which is the opposite of what should be done), causing an actual and sustained decrease in airspeed and then an engine stall.

While the odds of that plane crashing were at some point as insignificant as those of any other plane crashing, events transpired that increased those odds. When those young copilots were assigned to Flight 447, the odds grew. When the captain chose to go out the night before, the odds grew even more. When weather patterns changed and forced the airplane to fly through a storm, the odds grew to an insurmountable level.

Similarly, while the odds of Josh and me meeting might have been 0 percent at the moment of his birth, they changed over time. They increased when Vietnam revised its policy to permit those of ethnic Chinese ancestry to leave the country. They increased again when I made it to the refugee camps in Hong Kong. They increased dramatically when I set foot on American soil, and then again when I gained sight. They continued to increase as I chose to excel academically, as I ventured into uncharted territory by heading to the Northeast for college, as I stayed in New York after law school, as I chose to start my legal career at Cleary Gottlieb. They increased when Josh chose to be a tax lawyer, to do what very few from his community did and come to New York to practice the most exciting and challenging type of tax law, when he chose to accept a job offer at Cleary Gottlieb.

Numbers are not static. They are constantly changing, going up or down by degrees. Everyone agrees that with the outcome of my exploratory surgery, my odds of survival have increased. By how much? It's impossible to say. Josh has always told me that, much like the coming together of various random forces to cause an unlikely plane crash to occur or an unlikely pair like us to meet, in order for me to beat cancer, a series of things have to happen, like the falling of a row of dominoes.

Dr. D.L. agrees with Josh's view. Josh has told me from the beginning, "We need certain things to go our way." I needed to respond well to chemotherapy. I needed my CEA to be a reliable marker so as to warn me and my medical team about probable undetectable disease. I needed to have access to the best HIPEC surgeon possible. I needed to make some good decisions about if and when to undergo HIPEC and exploratory surgery. The disease in my peritoneum needed to respond to HIPEC. I needed an exploratory surgery to show no visible disease. All of those things happened. And then I had to find out that the "washings" tested negative for microscopic disease.

Of all that has gone right thus far, I've had very little control over anything. In general, beating cancer is about facts, circumstances, and occurrences that are uncontrollable (i.e., the extent of disease at diagnosis, access to health insurance and financial resources, capacity to understand and process medical information, emotional stamina, and most important of all, how a cancer's unique biology responds or doesn't respond to treatment).

Now the key is finding a way to make more dominoes fall, and the right way. But how do I do this when I have so little control? That is the question with which I am currently obsessed. I haven't spent much time basking in the joy of a clean surgery. I'm already thinking about the next move, trying to figure out what I can do to hold back this disease. Because in looking at the situation clearly, looking at those often-dynamic numbers, you realize that metastatic disease abides, and is resourceful. I haven't researched the likelihood of recurrence for me, but whatever it is, it's quite high, as it is for anyone with Stage IV disease. Dr. D.L. told Josh on Friday that the next three years are the critical period, that if I can hold back the disease during that time frame (even if I were to have a recurrence at some point afterward), my odds of long-term survival will increase significantly.

After I was first diagnosed, I asked my colorectal surgeon in a fit of desperation what I could do differently in terms of my personal choices to beat this disease, like exercising more than I had been (which was already a lot) or changing my diet, or taking supplements. He told me that when something like a cancer diagnosis happens, people try to find ways to control the disease in a world that seems to have gone crazy, but that anything a person could do would make very little difference.

In part, the answer to how I can make more dominoes fall is to re-dedicate myself to evaluating those things that *might* make a difference, however little. Since I have no control over the factors that will have a dramatic impact on my odds, then I will work at the margins on the theory that certain personal choices might lead to the critical tipping point. However, I am unwilling to subject myself to some life changes or financial expenditures without sufficient medical evidence. I intend to bury myself in research and studies in much the same way I once buried myself in school and legal work to determine for myself, notwithstanding the inconclusive evidence, whether a low-carb diet, cannabis oil, veganism, supplements, herbs, use of particular off-label drugs, maintenance chemo, experimental drugs, and other nonconventional treatments will make even a small difference by incrementally improving my odds of winning this war.

Beyond this, I can do nothing to make more dominoes fall. I must accept that I have no control over the factors that will really determine whether I live or die from this disease, that whether more dominoes fall is about God, faith, luck, prayer, hope, sheer randomness, or some combination of the above. And therein lies the intersection of Josh's science, studies, and statistics and my belief in those unquantifiable forces. If we can find the sweet spot in between those poles, I may beat this cancer yet.

Happy anniversary, darling.

21

Take Your Victories
Where You Can

After my clean MRI scan in early October, my oncologist, Dr. A.C., gave me four options: (1) continue with full-blown chemo, (2) go on maintenance chemo of 5-FU and Avastin, which inhibits the blood flow to cancer cells, but can also cause blood clots and hemorrhaging, (3) stop chemo altogether and proceed to a "wait-and-see" approach with monthly CEA testing and quarterly scans, or (4) take the rather unusual step of undergoing a "second-look" exploratory surgery to visually inspect my insides in what would be the most accurate and reliable form of monitoring (better than any scan). In light of the minimal risks involved, and the tremendous amount of information to be gained through Option 4, I decided to go with a second-look laparoscopy.

That surgery happened on Halloween Day 2014, and revealed that not only was I free from visible disease within the abdominal cavity, but based on the washings, or "cytology" in medical parlance (i.e., fluid flooded into the abdominal cavity, sucked out, and then tested), I was also free from microscopic disease, at least inasmuch as such a test could tell. It was not a result I or Dr. A.C. or my surgeon, Dr. D.L., expected. We were all prepared for the cytology to come back positive, so when it didn't, even though the results are only fifty-fifty reliable, we were all thrilled.

As Thanksgiving approached, I saw both Dr. A.C. and Dr. D.L., and they both hugged me, beaming. Dr. A.C. told me, "Good job," as if the outcome was something I had determined, and in that moment I felt his pride in me, not unlike a father's pride in his daughter. Implied in the hugs and the smiles from my doctors was a genuine delight in the victory we had won together, a self-satisfaction on their part with their technical skills and their compassionate humanity; a happiness, tinged with wonder, and a humble and grateful pride on my part—in the resilience of my body, a resilience that had by then allowed it to withstand the collateral damage of twenty-five rounds of chemotherapy and two surgeries. While I have often thought of how horrible and depressing it must be to be an oncologist, surgical or otherwise, I saw in my doctors' joy then how certain victories make it all worth it. With Stage IV disease, you take your victories where you can.

Dr. D.L. told me that what surprised him most about my surgery was not that my cytology had been negative but rather the remarkable absence of scar tissue, which had allowed him to see everything so clearly. Another person receiving the same HIPEC surgery (given the same history of a perforation at the time of the initial colon resection) would have likely developed significant amounts of scar tissue that would have made exploration difficult, forcing Dr. D.L. to maneuver the laparoscope every which way to see.

Scar tissue, also known as adhesions, is the frequent cause of bowel obstructions. Because the tissue can be as hard as cement, it also makes future surgeries, particularly laparoscopic ones, much more difficult. I had always understood that scar tissue starts to form the moment one's insides are exposed to air. Dr. D.L. said this is generally true. So why, I asked, had I not developed scar tissue? He said, maybe the postsurgical chemotherapy had inhibited the formation of scar tissue. But to tell the truth, he just didn't know. I think if he and I could unlock the mystery of why I escaped this common occurrence, we would both be quite famous and wealthy.

As I look at my paunchy stomach littered with ugly scars and deformed forever, a stomach that aggravates me to no end as it makes it so difficult for me to fit into my old clothes, I have to give it an affectionate pat—yes, I am proud of my body, this body that for some unknown reason resisted internal scarring, this body that despite everything it has been through remains fit and capable of keeping up (for the most part) with the twenty-something-year-old girls in their stylish tank tops and hip-hugging yoga pants at my gym. I am proud of my mind and spirit. I am proud of what I have achieved. I am grateful to have the doctors I have. I am grateful to have Josh, my girls, and the incredible support that surrounds me.

And yet, I understand that this is but a brief respite, an opportunity to regroup and strategize. I don't truly believe, notwithstanding the cytology results, that I am disease-free. Metastatic disease does not give up so easily, and I feel that there are inactive microscopic cancer cells inside of me.

Paradoxically, now that I am as clean as medical science can determine, returning to chemotherapy doesn't seem a viable option, as traditional chemotherapy attacks only active cancer, i.e., cancer that is multiplying. I am concerned with inactive cancer at this point, or cancer cells that are still in their infancy.

So, I set out to find new options for myself. I went to see Dr. Raymond Chang, a famous internist who specializes in nonconventional treatments. He is an MD, not a PhD or naturopath or other person claiming the title of medical doctor without legitimacy. I have met a couple of cancer patients who speak glowingly of him. Plus, my oncologist knows and likes him and even recommends him to his patients who are interested in integrative or alternative treatments. I read his book *Beyond the Magic Bullet,* which I thought was legitimate enough. In particular, I liked his strong emphasis on relying on human studies, as opposed to in vitro or animal studies. Based on all of the above, I was willing to go see him and pay the $875 an hour (which is not covered by insurance)—I try not to think of the money! (Incidentally, I've long since stopped taking the Chinese herbs from the Chinese medicine man because I didn't discern any noticeable effect, and I realized that I had become one of those people who was desperately grasping at straws without having done the research I needed to be comfortable.) In addition to vitamins and supplements and the like, Dr. Chang proposed alternatives like metronomic chemotherapy (i.e., delivering traditional chemo drugs at lower dosages but more frequently), hyperthermia (i.e., shooting the body with heated microwaves on the theory that the heat will kill tumors), and various non-FDA-approved drugs that are used in other countries and that he is able to import through the compassionate-use loophole in the federal laws. He did give me studies that accompanied every option he proposed and encouraged me to do my own reading. After some research and much thought, I've determined that the only thing I'm comfortable doing in the way of integrative and alternative therapies is vitamins and supplements (with limitations). I don't really believe those things will make much of a difference, but I think they will not harm me, so I'm willing to give them a try. I asked Dr. A.C. and Dr. D.L. their opinions, and they agreed with my conclusions. In fact, Dr. A.C. said the other stuff was "snake oil."

It's hard to avoid the talk of diets—whether vegan or alkaline or low carb—when you have cancer. Someone will inevitably say, You should juice or switch to a plant-based diet or avoid all sugars. People have asked me privately my opinion about diet, and I will state it here for the record. I tried a plant-based diet when I was first diagnosed—again one of those desperately grasping at straws acts—and I absolutely *hated* it. It's not that I love meat—in fact, I don't eat that much meat, and when I do it's mostly fish and poultry and organic at that—but I can't give up eggs, milk, butter, and cheese. Barring irrefutable evidence that animal products cause cancer, I'm not willing to give up certain things. The same is true of sugars and carbs. Food is a quintessential part of the human experience. The enjoyment of food is such a big part of life, and to give that up without the irrefutable evidence that might justify the sacrifice is a compromise in the quality of my life that I am unwilling to make. I believe in eating as much unprocessed food as possible, lots of fruits and vegetables and whole grains, with some meat and fish and the occasional dessert. I generally avoid red and smoked meats (although I do eat pork once in a while—we Chinese love our pork!). Everything in moderation, as they say.

Before my surgery, after I had asked online whether anyone had ever continued with full-blown chemo even with no evidence of disease (something my oncologist had favored at the time), a woman in one of my support groups sent me a private message. M is a researcher extraordinaire. She told me I might want to consider something called the ADAPT protocol, a treatment developed by Dr. Edward Lin out of the University of Washington that is currently in the Phase II clinical trial process. There are only three phases of testing before a drug is approved by the FDA, and Phase III is generally a rubber stamping, meaning much of the evidence in support of the drug therapy is established in the first two phases.

M sent me a link to the clinical trial at clinicaltrials.gov as well as links to the published journal articles discussing the results of the trials from 2007 through 2012. I read, and I made Josh read. The results in Phase II have been astounding—ninety-two-month survival rates for metastatic colon cancer for 40 percent of the cohort; this for a disease that typically sees an average of about twenty-four months. The protocol involves taking Xeloda, the oral form of 5-FU (which I've had all along), and Celebrex (an anti-inflammatory drug that is used to treat arthritis). Dr. Lin describes these drugs as working together to awaken the cancer stem cells and then kill them, akin to poking a beehive to bring out the bees and then spraying them with a pesticide. Dr. Lin likes to get patients to the point of no visible disease or as little visible disease as possible before starting this protocol, so it seems perfectly geared to someone in my position. I was persuaded.

I sent emails to both Dr. A.C. and Dr. D.L. before my appointments with them with links to the trial and the articles, letting them know that I would expect to hear their opinions. Both doctors think this is a reasonable next step for me, especially since they know that I'm not good at doing nothing. If I didn't do this protocol and I had a recurrence, I would kick myself a million times.

I have learned throughout this cancer journey that when the options aren't so appealing, you have to go out there and make new options. As much as I acknowledge how little control I have in my life, I do try to control what I can. Then I can let everything else go and let the universe do what it will.

22

The Cancer Is in My Lungs

It seems that the cancer wants to live, too.

In late December comes awful news.

I have about twenty 2- to 4-millimeter spots—also known as nodules—in my lungs. We are fairly certain they are cancer. The CT scan also shows that my right ovary is enlarged, which could be indicative of metastatic disease. If these are indeed cancer, then I am no longer curable, and my prognosis is, assuming I respond to chemo, "several years." That is the long and short of it.

No one went with me to see Dr. A.C. I went alone, and received the news alone. Which was probably for the best, as it allowed me time to cry alone, as I walked out, dazed, into a city all dressed up for Christmas. The thought of leaving my children and husband is unbearably painful. How will they go on without me? Who will pay the bills? Who will go to Costco to buy everything they need? Who will cook for them? Who will take the kids to school? Who will make their school lunches? Even as I think about going back on FOLFOX and enduring the horrible neuropathy, I have similar questions about how I and my family will get through the days, weeks, months, and years to come. And my parents . . . the thought of them watching me die breaks my heart anew. My sister told me she felt like we were back at square one.

No, I told her, it's worse than square one, because now it's in my lungs and I've already tried chemo regimens that haven't seemed to be that effective. In addition to having already tried the two leading chemo-therapy treatments for colorectal cancer, I am tired now, so tired of fighting, so tired of having any kind of hope and being painfully disap-pointed. I am so tired.

My instinct is to plan. I need to record for Josh how all our bills are paid every month so he will always keep the appropriate accounts funded. I need to figure out who is going to help raise my children, to make sure they take piano and swimming lessons, to make sure they learn to eat foods from all over the world, to keep the fridge and pantry stocked with the foods my husband and children love. I need to make memory books for the girls. I need to tell people how much I love them and let them know how they have affected my life. I need to extract promises from people to help look after my girls when I'm gone and for those who knew me best to tell my girls about me, to fill their ears with stories of me throughout all the phases of my life; I need those people to share with Mia and Isabelle what mattered to me most and the Chinese-rooted values that I hope my girls will learn. I need to take Josh and our girls to Disney World and the Ga-lápagos Islands so we can walk among hundred-year-old tortoises. I need to make a caramel soufflé like the heavenly one I ate with Josh in Paris last February. I need to scratch Josh's head just the way he likes it and to snuggle with my girls as much as I can. There is so much I need to do.

I know that soon I will regain my footing and I will get up and fight, that I will research and advocate for myself, that I will endure the treat-ments. But I also know that in order for me to suck the marrow out of what remains of my life, I need to acknowledge that I am now plan-ning for what is an inevitability. I must do all the things I have outlined. Josh has made me promise to fight, not to give up; he still clings to hope. But the most I can hope for now is time.

The sense that we ever had control over any of this seems nothing but a mockery now, a cruel illusion. And also, a lesson: we control nothing.

Well, that's not exactly true. We control how good we are to people. We control how honest we are with ourselves and others. We control the effort we have put into living. We control how we respond to impossible news. And when the time comes, we control the terms of our surrender.

2015

23

From Darkness to Strength

The day I got the horrible news, I learned of a laser surgery performed in Germany and London that is designed to deal with up to one hundred lung mets. Although the surgery has been performed for ten years, it is not available in the United States because the FDA has not approved the equipment. I asked my oncologist what he thought of the surgery and what his lung tumor board thinks. He says that my tumors are too small for the surgery, that a surgeon would not be able to see them to destroy them. What kind of war is this in which the lethal enemy won't show itself? Cancer fights dirty.

Dr. A.C. does have a patient he is sending to Germany to have it done, but he said that the surgeon would be able to *feel* her tumors. I might get a second opinion about this. The surgery costs eleven thousand euros per lung. Yikes!

I vowed when I started writing my way through this calamity that I would endeavor to be honest about who I am and what it is for me to battle cancer, that I would strive against my very human egoist tendencies to prop up some persona of myself as perpetually inspiring, strong, or wise. Why was this so important to me? In part because if this writing were to become the principal means by which my children would come to know my innermost thoughts and feelings after my death, I wanted them to see my real self, a self that, in addition to experiencing many moments of joy, gratitude, and insight, was often tormented by fear, anger, hurt, despair, and darkness. I also made that promise because I disliked tremendously those bloggers who always presented in the face of a life-threatening illness images of pumped fists and unending positivity and determination. To me, such portrayals were disingenuous, an insult to the intelligence of readers, and above all, disorienting and potentially harmful for those like myself who were newly diagnosed and felt more darkness than light. I wanted to detail and explore that darkness, to let others out there who I knew experienced a similar desolation and lonely darkness know that they were not and are not alone. There is a natural, intuitive fear of darkness; people who are gripped by it are ashamed to speak of it, while those who are free of it for however long wish to run from it as if it were a contagious plague. If the cost of my brutal honesty about my darkness is a highly unflattering picture of me that repels, so be it.

In the weeks after I received the news, I fell into a darkness that was a thousand times worse than anything I had experienced before. I managed to get through Christmas Day, and the full force of the darkness hit me the day after. It left me broken and crumpled on the ground, my rage-filled screams ringing in its wake and a husband and children utterly shocked at the madness they had never thought possible in this woman who was supposed to be their steadfast wife and mother.

Yes, Josh has seen me angry and despairing before, but never like this, for this frightened him; this made him afraid for his own and his children's safety, because I was like a deranged animal, devoid of reason, hope, and light. I yelled and hurled things, not at Josh or the children, but at the heartless gods who would do this to me and, in the absence of those gods, at the painfully unjust cruelty that is an inherent part of the human existence. Why me? I demanded of the gods. Hadn't I already borne my share of trials and tribulations? Hadn't I already known enough suffering? Hadn't I lived a good and moral life? The absence of any divine answer arising from the chaos of my thoughts made me even more crazed. Even the gods cower from me. Cowards.

Through heaving sobs, I begged Josh to let me go, to let me leave him and our girls forever, for all I wanted to do was flee, get on an airplane bound for unknown parts where I could die alone with a setting sun. In the state I was in, I was a completely unfit mother and wife, an unfit human being for that matter. I tried to convince Josh that my leaving would be for the best, that he is still a young, handsome man with a successful career and he would be able to find someone to replace me easily, that any woman would love our girls, that the girls are so young they would grow to love their new mother easily enough. I wanted not to fight, but to flee to a place where I could die. I told Josh I didn't want to live like this, with this diseased body that had failed me one time too many, with the specter of death looming ever closer; that this was no longer a life worth living, that whatever good that would come from now on, whatever laughter, whatever joy would be poisoned by the cancer, and I didn't want a life poisoned by cancer. I wanted to start over. I wanted to find escape and rebirth in death.

And then I grew angry at the image of this other woman who would have the time and life I should have had with Josh and my girls. I hate her, this woman I don't even know. I vow that if she does wrong by Josh and my children, I will hurt her. I will come back as a poltergeist and hurl books and vases and anything heavy and painful at her head. And yet I also want her, need her, to come into their lives, to take care of my husband and children. I need her to love them as well as if not better than I do; for as long as Josh and the girls are okay, then I know I will be okay. I need them to mourn me, to remember me for a time, and then I need them to move on and live their lives with joy and abandon. This is what I want for them above all else.

In sleep, I found a reprieve from my waking nightmare, for in sleep I do not have cancer. In sleep, I live the life I wanted. I've half convinced myself that death will be like my dreams. In death, my soul will travel to a different dimension, where I will get to live my ideal. There, I will no longer be plagued by the limitations and hurts of this body, but I will have the compassion and wisdom gained from the painful experiences of this life. There, I will know what it is like to see the world perfectly, to drive a car, fly a plane, play tennis. I will get to live a full and complete life with Josh, my great love of many lifetimes. With him, I will travel more of the world and have our two girls and more children. I will cook grand feasts for them and fill the house with the smell of freshly baked breads. Our home will ring with the sounds of innocuous yelling and mundane dramas and warm laughter. And there will be so much love, always so much love.

Every time I woke from sleep, the first thought I had was that I had incurable cancer with a prognosis of several years (and probably less given the seeming aggressiveness of the cancer), and I wanted to scream at the loss of my dreams in my waking hours. Each time I awoke was like mourning the loss of my dreams again and again and again. Torture. Agony. Crushing. It's enough to make you want to die so you can go live the life that you've half convinced yourself awaits.

Josh wouldn't allow me to lie broken on the ground. He yanked me up by the arms, screaming right back at me, "I will not let you give up. *Do you hear me?* You will not give up!" In the next breath, he was begging me to fight for him and the children, if not for myself.

I honestly think Josh and the girls would be better off starting over sooner rather than later. No one has been able to convince me otherwise. I don't want to be a burden. I don't want my family to see me die a slow and painful death. I don't want them to live through my emotional roller coaster. In no way am I minimizing the love Josh feels for me. It is very real and deep, but I also know that he is capable of loving someone else, that he should and will need to love someone else. And perhaps that love will be as profound as, if not more profound than, the love we have. He is a good and wonderful man, and I have been inordinately lucky to have him. And I know that the children are resilient, that they will withstand my loss and thrive regardless. They are, after all, my children, and I like to think the best of me flows through their veins.

I know that so many will step in to help Josh raise them and that so many will tell them about their mother. I know they will be surrounded by love.

So no, if I choose to keep fighting, it won't be because I think Josh and the girls really need me or that somehow more time with me will make much of a positive difference in their ultimate destinies. Nor will I fight based on some delusional hope that I will somehow still miraculously beat this, or that I will have a lot more time than I now expect to have. I have always had a tumultuous relationship with the concept of hope, and I still do. I'm not a believer. I will leave the hope stuff to all of you.

Even so, I do choose to keep fighting. It took me nearly two weeks to make that affirmative choice. It took me nearly two weeks to recover from the lows of that day after Christmas, to pull myself out of that darkness. It happened with the help of Josh and my girls, my beloved longtime therapist, and the words of my even more beloved sister, Lyna, and best friend, Sue. They helped me to see important truths about me and how I want my life to be viewed now and after I am gone.

When I did poorly on a test in high school—and by "poorly" I mean by my nerdy standards a 92 instead of a 95, or a 97 instead of 100—I would come home tearful, convinced that this unacceptable grade was the greatest tragedy of my young life, and indeed it was. My parents were not the typical crazy Asian American parents who put pressure on us. Yes, my dad would pay us for every A we got on our report cards, but there were never any demands or threats. In response to my crying, my mother would ask in her broken English, "Did you do the best you can?" Of course I had. "Then that's all you can do," she would tell me.

It was such simplistic advice, and yet it was so true. Your best effort is all you can ask of yourself—no more and no less. And once you've done that, there can be no regrets. I will continue to fight this disease—not with the same gung-ho attitude I had at the beginning—but I will continue to fight it with an even more nuanced, deeper, and more realistic understanding of its deadliness. I am an overachiever, used to doing my best at everything. A lot of times my best wasn't good enough to get the stellar grades. Similarly, my best will not be enough to beat cancer, but even as I lie dying someday not that far in the future, to know that I tried my best to gain more time in this life and to live as well as possible in the face of this disease and therefore have no regrets, that knowledge will be enough for me. It will bring me peace, because by choosing to fight without ceasing, even in the face of such a formidable foe, I will teach my girls one of the most important lessons there can be. I want them to understand the importance of always doing the best they can in whatever endeavor, a lesson that their maternal grandmother taught me and one that I now must teach them.

As a mother, I don't get to just walk away from my children, however much I may want to escape further physical and emotional pain or for any other selfish reasons. I made the choice to be a mother and with that choice came sacrosanct commitments, the most important among them being to give my children the tools to live their lives, tools that go well beyond feeding, bathing, and clothing them. Continuing to live and battle this disease in the face of its likely outcome is about keeping the most sacred promises I made to them on the days I held each of their little, fragile bodies in my arms for the first time.

And, by God, I will live with joy.

After the bad news, I received many wonderful messages of support and love, from intimates as well as strangers. All of them lifted my spirit, and got me thinking that somehow my fight was also their fight, and the notion that I must continue to fight for them was incredibly beautiful to me, and in turn gives me the will to fight even more.

It is as John Donne wrote in his "no man is an island" meditation: "Any man's death diminishes me, because I am involved in mankind." Yes, I suppose that my death will diminish you, but I also understand now that my living and fighting makes you greater than you are. We humans are resilient little bugs. And indeed, anyone who chooses to live and fight and show by example the power of the human spirit that we all share, and its determination to persevere against the brutalities of what life can bring, strengthens us all with a sense of the tremendous potential and fortitude that lie within each of us, a potential that is realized only when truly tested.

So I fight for myself, for my family, for the message that my war against cancer conveys to all of you, to all of humanity, about the incredible strength of which we are all capable. And by that same token, I urge all of you who face your own challenges that make you want to fall into the darkness to fight, too, because you, too, are part of humanity, and your fight matters and gives me and others strength when we falter.

As the new year began, I received many messages reminding me of how brave and strong I am. Which in the moment felt akin to telling a

Chihuahua that he is actually Great Dane. I felt anything but brave and strong during those weeks. Does a brave and strong person lie on the ground crying as her children look on in horror? No, those are not images of bravery and strength. It is what she does afterward, though, that matters. A brave and strong person then hugs her daughters and tells them stories about her childhood, and even though they're too young to understand, she talks to them about what it means to get married one day and how important it is for them to love themselves first and foremost before thinking about loving someone else. A brave and strong person pulls herself out of the abyss with the help of those who have more strength, hope, and faith than she and goes about the business of living even though she doesn't necessarily want to. A brave and strong person goes back to doing more research as she tries to figure out what to do next. She does all this knowing that there will be another abyss and many more moments and hours and days of darkness before she succumbs to the inevitable.

24

"Keeping It in the Stomach"

Enough gloom and doom from me.

Who's got time for that?

I need to resolve something here. I want to talk about love, and about other words, spoken and unspoken. I want to talk about my mother and my grandmother. My grandmother—*that* grandmother—the larger-than-life woman whom I had loved so completely and respected so much for her intelligence and indomitable strength. When she died so suddenly of colon cancer at the age of seventy-three, I was convinced that I would suffocate beneath the weight of all the grief, for it was the first time in my twenty years of life that someone I loved and someone I believed loved me just as much had left me.

But then, when my mother told me how much my grandmother had loathed me, I had to learn to hate, because I wanted to hate her back—this woman who was a stranger to me now—with as much venom as she had shown me, and to set fire to everything good I had ever thought of or felt for her. I wanted to yank her back from the spirit world to demand that she answer for her crimes against me, for her betrayal.

In the aftermath of that initial eruption was a scorched terrain of deep, inconsolable hurt and an insatiable need to know if she and the rest of them had ever loved me or been sorry for what they all had tried to do, if any of them ever shuddered at the idea of their daughter/ granddaughter dead before she had a chance to live. Was that why my father had suddenly cried upon seeing me trying on my black cap and gown the day before my college graduation, tears rolling down his roughened cheeks in a way that struck me as too much and too odd for that occasion, no matter how proud he might have been? Was he sorry then, wordlessly apologizing to me with every tear? What had my grandmother been thinking in that picture of her holding my hand in the perfectly manicured gardens at the Huntington Library when I was seven years old, wearing pigtails and my Buddy Holly glasses? Or what about when she sat down next to me and patted me on the back in that restrained, affectionate manner that was her way when I got my period for the first time? She'd seemed so proud. Was that the same woman who ten years earlier had been so concerned with what would happen to me when I started menstruating, horrified at the thought of me bleeding everywhere like a wild animal?

Did you think then about how you had wanted to put me to sleep like some rabid dog?

After the hurt came the need to clear the smoke and ashes so I could move on (I am moving on still), to create order out of the chaos in my mind, with rationalization and even pity for these misguided people I had to call my family. They were all superstitious souls trapped in a backward, hopeless country, trying to survive in difficult times, living within a culture where female infanticide was not an unfamiliar idea. Perhaps in that situation, even *I* would have thought murder was justified . . . perhaps.

Don't fool yourself. You know you wouldn't have. Even the herbalist, who by the way came from the same time and place as all of them, knew that.

I could definitely feel sorry for my mother, if no one else. She was the biggest victim. Yes, she was beautiful, but she was fearful and lacked the assertive personality needed to challenge my domineering grandmother. She had been taught to be respectful of and obedient to her elders and to quash her own selfish voice for the selfless good of the family. It was easy for me to imagine my mother cowering before my grandmother's will, because all through my childhood I witnessed my mother fleeing from confrontations at home and at work. My frequently ill-tempered father cursed and yelled at her whenever he felt like it for silly and sundry things—rinsing the dishes twice because she was neurotically afraid of us ingesting detergent or watching the water boil for soup when she should have been more efficient by prepping the vegetables for the soup—to the point where I wanted to throw my little, meaty body over her thin one to shelter her from his verbal daggers. Exasperated, I once asked her why she never fought back against my father or that co-worker who had maligned her in front of everyone at work but whom she condemned in turn only in the confines of our home.

She said it was better to "keep it in the stomach," a Vietnamese phrase that means to hold one's tongue, to keep it bottled up inside, all for the sake of preserving the peace. Even as she revealed the truth to me almost thirty years after it all happened and almost ten years after my grandmother's death, she was still nervous, afraid of breaking the pact of secrecy that had held them together for all those years, a pact that had become severely weakened in the absence of my grandmother's silencing presence.

"If your grandmother were still alive, I would not tell you what I am about to tell you, and your grandfather and your father will yell at me until the end of my life or theirs if they find out," she said as she began the story. Her eyes, brows, and mouth had pulled into a rigid mask as if to defend against the inevitable attacks. Yet she was willing to take the risk to tell me.

She said she told me because I had the right to know. She was right. I did have the right to know. But I don't believe that was the only reason for her.

True to her belief in "keeping it in the stomach," my mother is adept at repressing her darker emotions. I can remember her crying only twice in my presence—once at my grandmother's funeral, where she suddenly burst into tears, and the other time as she said goodbye to me in my college dorm room right before the beginning of freshman year, when she was blinking so much that I thought her eyelashes might fall off. While words flow easily to her when telling any story, they seem to dry up when they could be used to expose her vulnerability.

In my family she is not alone in that regard. Words like "I'm sorry" or "I love you" or even "thank you" are never uttered in my family, although there are exceptions among those of my generation who grew up in America. Otherwise, those types of words are simply not part of our spoken familial language. Instead, we are forced to interpret the words that are spoken to us and to master an unspoken language in which our actions are our words.

When my parents cook my favorite dishes in the whole world in honor of my visits home, they are showing me how much they love me, which has always struck me as a much more compelling and persuasive expression of love than simply saying words.

So even though my mother seemed to tell the story without emotion that night, I knew that below the surface there were so many unspoken messages, things that my mother wanted me to know but she just couldn't bring herself to say aloud. Later I would mull over the music in her voice, the nuance behind her every word, and the subtlety of her body language a thousand times, maybe a million times, to figure it all out. In the slightly elevated pitch of her voice, almost angry sounding, somewhat akin to that of a petulant child denying responsibility for something, and in the even slighter jutting of her chin, there was defensiveness against the reproach she expected from me. *It wasn't my idea. I didn't really want to do it,* she seemed to be saying. Mostly, though, there was guilt. Her defensiveness would not have existed but for the guilt.

I knew based on statements she'd made over the years that she felt responsible for my being born with cataracts, statements like "I was stupid to take those pills while I was pregnant with you." She is the type of woman who sucks blame and guilt into herself through a giant straw. She would say things like "I couldn't find any cow's milk for you when you were a baby. You would have been so much taller if I had been able to." It was her fault that my skin was too dark because she hadn't known the right foods to feed me. It was her fault that I didn't get into Yale since she hadn't pushed me hard enough.

If my mother was going to feel guilt for the cataracts and things like my height and the color of my skin and the fact that I couldn't quite make it into Yale, then the guilt she carried for taking me to see that herbalist must have been unbearable. For twenty-eight years my mother had tried to repress the guilt of attempting to kill me, and that night she finally stopped trying. In the very act of telling me, of risking my father's and grandfather's wrath, of freeing herself from the frightened woman she has always been, of finding the courage to look me in the eye and admit what she had done, she was begging me for absolution, giving me the power to free her from her guilt.

Absolution is difficult. Sometimes it just isn't possible. Pity is one thing. Forgiveness is something else altogether.

That night, those words, "Please forgive me," unspoken, hung between my mother and me after she had finished telling her story and after she asked me to not tell anyone what I had just learned. She stood over me with her hands at her sides, waiting. I could not look at her. At some point during her telling of the story—I don't know when—I had begun to weep. I am not like the other members of my family. I am not good at holding back my tears, suppressing my emotions. I left her room then, feeling enlightened, angry, hurt, confused, sad, but mostly battered, knowing that I would never look at my family, my life, or myself in quite the same way again. Before I left my mother, I thanked her for telling me because I truly was grateful.

It's better to know than not know.

25

A Day in My Life

After I graduated from law school, in 2002, I went to work at Cleary Gottlieb, a prominent international law firm, what you would have called a Wall Street law firm back in the day, the kind of firm that represents the great American blue-chip companies and investment banks in their many million- and billion-dollar corporate transactions and lawsuits, which more often than not make the headlines of *The Wall Street Journal*. Many law school students graduating from the big-name schools work for a few years at a big law firm to pay off school debt and get some experience before heading out to do other things—work for themselves, or take a job with the government, a nonprofit, a smaller firm, or a corporation as an in-house counsel. A small minority have the stamina, desire, and talent to actually vie for a coveted place among the illustrious partnerships of these traditional law firms.

I stayed longer at Cleary than I ever thought I would, and was still there when I was diagnosed. I was not on the partnership track, as I certainly lacked the stamina and talent to be a partner. After years of slaving away, pulling all-nighters, and living under the intense stress of being an associate at a place like Cleary, I had finally found a comfortable niche that was somewhat conducive to being a mother to young children. And then cancer struck.

I haven't worked since I was diagnosed. As varied as my days were in the law, it's even more remarkable to me now how no day in my life is ever the same. I have no set schedule other than getting the girls ready for, and taking them to, school every morning, and putting them to bed every night. In between, I cook, clean, write, read, research, talk to cancer and noncancer friends, watch TV, occasionally hang out with people, pay bills, fundraise for colorectal cancer research, and stare at the ceiling. I honestly have no idea where all the time goes, a scary thought considering how limited my time is.

I applaud all those who work while living with active Stage IV disease and even more so those who have young children; I know not working is often not an option; nonetheless, I admire those people's ability to juggle work on top of the emotionally and physically draining life that is living with cancer.

On a Monday in early January 2015, when the news of my sobering prognosis was still fresh and painful, I woke up before dawn on the wrong side of the bed. I was plagued by doubts and questions for which I did not have the answers. Should I experiment with cannabis oil? Should I be adding or removing certain supplements? Should I be seeking a second opinion? Should I see another oncologist altogether, someone who specializes in colorectal cancer, someone at the esteemed Memorial Sloan Kettering? Should I be more aggressively pursuing laser surgery in Germany despite my oncologist's and the lung tumor board's opinion? That morning, for whatever reason, the worries were overwhelming.

My younger daughter, three-year-old Isabelle, also seemed to have woken up out of sorts. The darkness outside seemed to match the darkness within us both. Monday mornings during the winter are particularly painful with the kids as I struggle to get them out the door, knowing that we'll be late, but still striving to arrive within some acceptable limits of tardiness for kindergarten and nursery school. But that Monday morning was exceptionally painful. Isabelle was especially challenging in her refusal to cooperate and in her extreme clinginess to me. When she becomes unusually clingy, I always think she knows something that I don't, that she can sense the cancer growing

inside me. She was like that in December in the weeks before my troubling CEA test and damning scan.

I kept telling Josh that Isabelle sensed the growth of metastatic disease in me, but he told me I was being ridiculous, that such behavior
could be attributable to any number of things. Of course, I was right.

I always think of Mia as my stunningly beautiful and intellectual
child, the kind of girl who will turn—and has already turned—heads
with her captivating face and tall grace, and who astounds as she points
to an animal in a medieval painting in a museum and declares, "That's
the narwhal, the unicorn of the sea." While I fear she may battle her
own demons born of innate insecurity one day, Mia is my adventurous
eater and the one who I suspect will follow in my footsteps in learning
multiple languages and traveling to the far reaches of the world.

But Belle (who is more stubborn than a mule—she would rather
starve and faint than eat what she doesn't want to eat, for instance) is
my ageless soul, my uncannily intuitive child, who understands people
and life with a precociousness well beyond her years. She is my child
who talks to ghosts. When she had just turned two and a half, as I was
pushing her off the elevator in her stroller one morning, out of no-
where she asked me, "What happens when we die, Mama?" I didn't
know how to respond, for I would never have expected that kind of
question from a two-and-a-half-year-old child.

It was also around that time that Mia was being especially difficult—so difficult that I felt like she and I were already having those
raging fights I've heard occur between mothers and their teenage
daughters; my mother and I didn't fight like that. One Sunday night,
Mia had pushed me over the brink and I let loose on her, yelling and
ordering her to her room. She went running, tears streaming down her
cheeks and screams echoing with the slam of the door. I cried hysterically on the couch, beating myself up for being the worst mother ever.
Josh told me to retreat to our room so Isabelle wouldn't have to see me
so upset—he thought my crying would scare her. In response, Belle
turned to her father and declared in her sweet voice, "Mama is just really tired now. She's gonna cry for a little bit and then she will be okay."

During my illness, the children have witnessed my emotional

outbursts—the crying, the screaming, the rage. I'm sure many child psychologists believe that Josh and I should hide our emotions and the truth from our children, that they are fragile flowers that should be protected. Josh and I don't subscribe to that thinking. We do not believe in hiding from our children. They are not fragile flowers that will wilt under the strain; rather, they are highly intelligent little girls with an enormous capacity to understand and grow stronger with every hard reality that awaits them in their lives. Facing hardship with a solid foundation of familial love from an early age will strengthen them. I know this to be true based on my own life.

When I lie in bed crying, Mia usually stays away, or she'll run into my room to grab her stuffed animal Pinky and her blanket and run right out to watch TV—she internalizes her fears, worries, and sadness. Belle, on the other hand, comes to check on me every couple minutes, opening the door ever so quietly to stick her head inside to look at me with her concerned brown eyes. Sometimes, she crawls into bed with me and gives me a hug and kiss. "Mommy, it's going to be okay," she reassures me, like she knows all.

But on that particular Monday morning, Belle was not the reassuring voice she sometimes is. I cried into her neck as she sat on my lap in the hallway outside her classroom. We have to kill thirty minutes every morning between 8:30, when Mia's class starts, and 9:00, when Belle's class starts. I sat there on the floor listening to other parents cheerily greeting each other and comparing notes about their holidays as if they didn't have a care in the world. Our holidays had been awful, completely poisoned by cancer. At that moment, the sounds of normalcy were more than I could handle. In our little corner, I tried to hide as I sobbed, holding Belle even tighter. There were no questions or other words this time, no "Mommy, why are you crying?" or "Mommy, it's going to be okay." Instead, she just sat staring at a spot on the wall with that look in her eyes that told me she was seeing something I couldn't see, in a place to which I could not go with her, the look that scares me because I know she knows that there is worsening metastatic disease.

Her silence ended in the classroom as we tried to part for the day. I was still crying, thinking of all the school dropoffs I will miss in the years to come. I was gripped by an overwhelming sense of the futility of everything, that no matter what I did I was going to die from this disease, that it was simply a matter of time, probably less time rather than more, and that this little girl would be deprived of the person who loves her most. She was now fighting for me to stay with her. "Don't go, Mommy! *Don't go!*" she begged. I needed one of the assistant teachers to pry her out of my arms so I could leave, running out of the room, afraid to look back while her cries rang in my ears.

As I left the school, I begged whatever gods there may be for a sign, a sign that my efforts to fight this disease and thus the rest of my life would not be futile, that this misery that had come for me was not going to completely choke the life out of me, that I could still derive some untarnished happiness from life, that I would find some peace amid all the doubts that cluttered my mind. You know you're really in the depths of despair when you start begging the gods for signs.

As I began the twenty-minute walk north on Court Street toward the Trader Joe's—I needed to do a quick grocery run before heading in for my next treatment—I heard someone call my name. I turned, embarrassed at my obvious distraught state, as a woman I didn't recognize approached me.

"We're here to help," she said. "Please let us know how we can help."

I was even more embarrassed at my inability to place this woman—facial recognition has never been one of my strengths, due to my poor vision. She was one of Isabelle's classmates' mothers. She and others knew about my situation. The class parents wanted to help. I was so touched. I told her there wasn't anything in particular at that moment, but that I was keeping track of all offers, for there would be a time when I would need as much help as I could get. I started crying, and she cried with me, and we stood in the middle of the broad sidewalk hugging. Was this my sign from the gods?

After buying the groceries and hauling them home on the B63 bus down Atlantic Avenue, I put lidocaine cream on the skin covering the mediport in my chest in preparation for the giant needle that would be inserted an hour later and hopped on the subway toward the NYU Cancer Center. I was walking east on Thirty-fourth Street, glumly lost in my own thoughts, when a petite but plump black-haired woman, probably in her fifties, approached me with a piece of paper. Great. Now what? I thought she was going to solicit money from me. The woman didn't speak much English, but she managed to convey to me that she needed directions and handed me the slip of paper. It contained written directions to the NYU Cancer Center. How ironic.

"I'm going there, too. Just follow me," I said, oddly buoyed by the knowledge that I wasn't the only one heading to that dreaded place.

"What kind of cancer do you have?" I asked. Have you figured out by now that I'm nosy and will ask all those personal questions of strangers that most people would never ask? She pointed to her breasts.

"I have colon cancer," I told her, pointing to my lower abdomen.

Based on the confused expression on her face, I wasn't confident she entirely understood me, so I asked, "Do you speak Spanish?" just in case I could communicate with her better in my terrible Spanish.

She shook her head.

"Where are you from?" I asked, carefully enunciating every syllable.

"Bangladesh," she said.

Now, that was really weird. How many people do you encounter from Bangladesh, even in a diverse city like New York? I think I've met only one other person from Bangladesh in New York City in all my years living here. What's more, Bangladesh has a particular significance to me. I lived there for ten weeks the summer after my first year in law school, interning at a local human-rights nongovernmental organization. The experiences I had during those ten weeks were among the most enriching and profound of my life. My time there was fraught with all the discomfort of living amid extreme heat, monsoons, untilthen-unimaginable poverty, and cultural displacement, and the pain of observing girl prostitutes living in squalor and women with their noses burned off by sulfuric acid thrown at them by their abusive husbands. But my time there was also filled with the self-knowledge and pride that I could endure and even thrive with discomfort, finding wonder and gratitude in the unmatched beauty and richness of a lush and unspoiled countryside and the unparalleled kindness and resilience of the people.

As I looked at this Bangladeshi woman who had chosen me to ask for directions, all the associations I have with Bangladesh—the juxtaposition of ugliness and beauty, suffering and joy, poverty and generosity—came back to me. My journey through cancer is not so different from my journey through Bangladesh; this cancer journey has been and is one filled with ugliness and beauty, suffering and joy, poverty and generosity. How could I help but think that this Bangladeshi woman's momentary visit in my life was not random at all?

26

Invincibility

Every time I see Dr. A.C., my vital signs are measured by Tanya. Tanya is an outspoken, middle-aged black woman and mother of two, who likes to wear scrubs printed with different cartoon characters. Like beacons of cheer and light in a place that can be so grim, her scrubs have always entertained me as I expectantly wait to see what character it will be this time. We talk about cartoons, our kids, our vacations, and sometimes we gossip about the staff and even Dr. A.C., because, as I've said, I'm very nosy. Such conversations with the various people I encounter at the NYU Cancer Center—Tanya, the receptionists, the nurses, Dr. A.C. himself—lift my spirits; they make me feel like these people care about me and I about them, like they don't view me as just a cancer patient but as a vital, involved, invested, and interested member of the human race who is more than just her cancer. I think most people would be surprised at how much I laugh in the cancer center.

It was during one of these conversations with Tanya that I asked casually, "So, you must see really sick people here." Of course, I had noticed in my frequent stints in the waiting room that I was invariably one of the youngest people there, that I indeed, despite my diagnosis and prognosis, most often looked the healthiest.

Tanya lowered her voice into a conspiratorial whisper. "Oh, yeah.

Some people come in looking like they're two days away from death asking for treatment, or a second or third or fourth opinion."

I was shocked. "Seriously?" In my many hours of hanging out in the waiting room and the exam rooms during the past twenty-one months, not so subtly checking out my fellow cancer patients out of the corner of my eye—or really, most often I stare—I had never seen anyone who looked that sick.

She nodded solemnly.

At my following visit, as I was leaving the exam room in which I had just met with Dr. A.C., an EMT was wheeling into my room a sickly old man with a few strands of wispy white hair. He lay there, on a stretcher, unmoving. Tanya rushed in to take his vitals, slamming the door as I made a narrow escape. She hadn't been exaggerating! People who are very ill from cancer go to the ER or the hospital to address symptoms or complications; they don't come to visit the oncologist in his office unless they want treatment or an opinion.

There was something disquieting about that man, about all the other patients near death who come to Dr. A.C.'s office and the offices of thousands of other oncologists in this country and throughout the world. More disturbing to me was the thought of the many others who go to see pseudodoctors and blatant charlatans in Mexico and Germany and South Africa or even New York City who prey on the desperately sick with their highly questionable treatments at the cost of hundreds of thousands of dollars and untold physical suffering. Not to mention the emotional trauma at the inevitable failure of such quackery. In the hope of physical salvation, people will spend their last dollars and last days drinking green sludge drawn from a swamp and filling their veins with a clear liquid of who the hell knows what. Desperate people go looking for miracles, and there is a shady industry that caters in said "miracles."

I have told my good friend X—or maybe more truthfully I vowed to X—"I will never be one of those people; I will never go to Mexico to drink sludge, no matter what happens." My friend, this brilliant man with a razor-sharp intellect, replied, "I think I would be one of those people." I was appalled, horrified, perplexed, and also intrigued by his response. Why indeed would someone so smart do something so dumb? X doesn't have cancer. Even so, in the cancer world, I've seen quite a bit of that—sick people doing crazy things in order to save themselves, and some of them I would say are quite mentally competent and even smart under other circumstances. (Consider, as an example of someone brilliant robbed of rationality, Steve Jobs, who rejected conventional treatments in favor of alternative treatments at a time when his pancreatic cancer was very treatable; even though he subsequently underwent surgery and other traditional therapies, many consider his initial rejection of conventional care to have shortened his life.)

Something about cancer—in which the machine of our very existence, cellular reproduction, turns against us—makes us humans crazed. It is easy to see how that creates within our flawed selves irrationality, fanaticism, and desperation.

Should desperate people be commended for their bravery, for fighting against all odds, for leaving no stone unturned, for "raging against the dying of the light" until their absolute last breath, despite the debilitating consequences of treatment, for staying put in the face of a destructive hurricane and saying a symbolic "fuck you" to the cruel fates? Should I praise them in the same way I praise a woman who chooses to endure the pain of childbirth without an epidural—I screamed for an epidural the moment my contractions started—or a man who survives at sea with little food and water? Early on in my cancer journey, I vowed that I would be one of them—that I would forever rage against the dying of the light. Back then, maybe I would have considered seeking chemotherapy treatment days before my death and even drinking sludge. No longer.

I've had my moments of irrationality, fanaticism, and desperation, too, of course. Moments that I now view with some degree of embarrassment. I've paid a total of eighteen hundred dollars to see the famed integrative doctor Raymond Chang. I've spent thousands of dollars on supplements, herbs, and cannabis, based on Dr. Chang's recommendations or on the Internet success story du jour, or whatever link someone shared on some forum. Other than vitamin D, CoQ10, and Cimetidine, all of the supplements now sit on my kitchen counter untouched. (I never seriously entertained Dr. Chang's more drastic treatment proposals, such as hyperthermia and immunotherapy-like treatments available only in other countries.) At my last infusion, I told Dr. A.C. (who has always been okay with me taking supplements), that I've stopped taking all the things Dr. Chang recommended because ultimately I just don't believe, and I can't do something I don't believe in. Dr. A.C. responded, "You don't believe because at heart you are a scientist." I think that was the greatest compliment Dr. A.C. could have paid me. I've always been skeptical of alternative treatments, but skepticism turned to disbelief when after my recurrence Dr. Chang recommended scorpion venom at six hundred dollars for a month's supply. I went home and watched the *Nightline* story about scorpion venom, which basically called it snake oil.

The hope industrial complex won't get another dime out of me. Or rather, the industrial complex that preys on the hopeful will get no more support from me.

Many advocates of alternative treatments make the common argument that anything is worth trying so long as no harm is done. This is the same basis upon which my own oncologist acquiesces to his patients doing alternative treatments—that so long as the treatments do not negatively impact organ function, he will allow them. He is skeptical, of course, but I suspect he recognizes that many of his patients crave control over their destinies (ha!) and must feel as if they are leaving no option unexplored. Even though he and other scientifically minded people understand that control is an illusion, I suppose that illusion can be important to the preservation of a dying patient's sanity.

But a beating heart alone does not make for a life. So what was that old man searching for on that stretcher, and what would X want if he ever got to that point? I wonder. A miracle? A cure? More time? To prove his own resilience? *What?* Is there some base primal instinct compelling them to fight for survival at any cost, like a wild animal clawing savagely against its natural predator? Are they that afraid of death? Or do they love life that much? Or are they weighed down by the obligations of love that dictate they must live as long as possible under any circumstance for those who rely on them? What motivates them, fear or love, death or life? I've been pondering these questions deeply since that conversation with Tanya, trying to determine how I would answer them as I make decisions about whether and how to live what remains of my days.

I suspect that the old man and X, like many people, are more afraid of death than they are in love with life, and that an animalistic fear overrides whatever rational intelligence they possess; I would guess that they fear the unknown of what Shakespeare called the "undiscovered country," the probable nothingness they believe lies beyond this life despite their wavering belief in God; they fear having the fire of their existence extinguished as if they had never been; they fear being small and irrelevant and forgotten. I've seen people only days from death proclaim to a mostly unbelieving audience on social media how they're still going to beat their cancer. I read somewhere that those people who cling to such unrealistic hopes have egos that cannot fathom their own nonexistence, the very notion so incomprehensible, so incongruous with everything that has ever been their reality, so wrong that their minds must reject, reject, and reject until there can no longer be denial of what in fact is objective reality.

It seems I don't have much of an ego (at least not the kind of ego that clings to its own existence)—my Freudian therapist would know better than I—for I don't have such a powerful fear of what awaits in the undiscovered country, perhaps because I do believe there is another country and not just nothingness. I can't explain to you why I believe; it is simply a matter of intuition and faith. For me, death waits like a doorway beckoning me to a new adventure, yet another on my long list of adventures, a new territory to explore and understand and from which my everlasting soul will learn and evolve.

I don't want to mislead in suggesting that I don't have an ego—we all do—a place in which our arrogance and conceit are born. My ego thrives on a belief in, and the need to continually cultivate, my inner strength and courage, my innate sense of grace and dignity that has heretofore allowed me to withstand the vicissitudes of life with a sometimes brutal self-honesty, and then to arise after shouting the expletives and shedding the tears, smiling and laughing at myself. I've never been a beauty, nor have I ever been the smartest person at school or work, but because of the circumstances of my life and the successes

I have achieved despite those circumstances, I have always believed myself to be strong and resilient. I am good at looking directly at the harshness of life's reality. I have faith and pride in my own spiritual invincibility.

I couldn't say it better than Albert Camus, who wrote:

> In the midst of winter, I found there was, within me, an invincible
> summer.

And that makes me happy. For it says that no matter how hard the world pushes against me, within me, there's something stronger—something better, pushing right back.

For me, raging and raging like a wild, irrational beast, denying one's own mortality, clinging to delusion and false hopes, pursuing treatment at the cost of living in the moment, sacrificing one's quality of life for the sake of quantity, none of this is graceful or dignified, and all of it denies us our contemplative and evolved humanity; such acts do not cultivate an invincible spirit; such acts are not testaments to inner strength and fortitude. For me, true inner strength lies in facing death with serenity, in recognizing that death is not the enemy but simply an inevitable part of life.

Ever since I learned that my cancer had metastasized to my lungs and that I have a dim prognosis, more than one person has commented on a change in me, and on my resigned tone, as if I have accepted my death from this disease as a foregone conclusion, even if I don't know when exactly that will be. More than one person has told me that I seem to have lost my traditional fierceness. Even Josh accuses me now of being a defeatist, that by conceding my fate, I am succumbing to the disease, that I have stopped fighting.

Josh and others have misinterpreted my actions. It is true—I have spent the last few months confronting my mortality, accepting the likelihood of my death from my cancer, trying to find peace with my destiny. But what Josh and others don't understand is that with acceptance and peace, I have learned to live more fully and completely in the here and now, that I now live with a fierceness, passion, and love that I've never known. In what is the greatest irony of all, I have come to realize that in accepting death, I am embracing life in all of its splendor, for the first time. Indeed, the part of me that believes in things happening for a reason believes that I am, through this cancer journey, meant to understand within the depths of my soul this paradox of death and life.

With that in mind, Josh and I planned a trip. On July 2, we will leave for Quito, the capital of Ecuador, where we will stay for less than two days, visiting the old colonial town (a UNESCO World Heritage Site), and on July 4, we will fly to an island in the Galápagos archipelago, where we will board a thirty-two-person yacht that will serve as our home for the next eight days. The yacht will motor from island to island by night, and by day we will hike, snorkel, and kayak in places that few have ever been, where prehistoric-looking animals roam free, having been largely undisturbed for centuries. Josh and I are looking at it as the trip of our lifetime together.

I don't visit cancer support group sites very much anymore. I don't research alternative treatments anymore. Alternative treatments require a fair amount of energy to research and to generally pursue, and that for me detracts from my ultimate objective of living in the moment. I don't research conventional treatments much either these days. I'm honestly too busy living, too busy spending time with my family, too busy cooking, too busy pursuing a huge project that involves the expansion of our home. The time will come when I will have to focus once again on cancer, on clinical trials, on choosing new therapies, but the time is not now. Now, even as death lurks all around me, I live fully and completely while I am relatively healthy and pain-free; now I suck the marrow out of this glorious life I have been given.

That all being said, nothing is ever so simple, is it?

When I went to see Dr. A.C. to discuss the possibility of changing treatment (i.e., switching to something more aggressive that might actually shrink my tumors—as opposed to just maintaining the status quo—at the cost of my quality of life), without Josh present, I expressed to him my wishes. "I want to be clear that I am not one of those people who wants to cling to life by a fingernail, that I will always choose quality over quantity, that facing death with dignity and grace means more to me than adding days to my life on this planet," I declared. But then I paused. I voiced next what I had not verbalized before. "But in telling you this, I feel like I am betraying my husband and little girls, that for them I should choose to live as long as possible at any cost to myself, that time with them is priceless."

What will my children think of me one day? How will they judge me? Will they call me a defeatist, too? Will they resent me for not fighting harder, for not expending more energy on figuring out ways to extend my life? Would they admire me more as a woman who lived well in spite of her disease or would they respect me more if I were like that old man being wheeled into an oncologist's office? Would I be setting a better example for them if I raged or if I went quietly into that good night? I don't know the answers to these questions. And I don't know whether those answers should really influence my decisions about my own life. All I know is that I love my daughters.

Hours after I'd expressed my sentiments to Dr. A.C., my sister came over to take the girls to Target to pick up a Mother's Day gift for me. I did not go with them. My sister later recounted how she instructed Isabelle to pick a card for me (not that the child can yet read). Belle sat in the shopping cart and pointed to one card and one card alone, screaming that she chose that one. When they came home, my sister handed me the card adorned with a golden butterfly and told me that Isabelle alone had chosen it. Of course, it would be Isabelle who selected a card out of hundreds that had such meaning, as if she knew what thoughts I had been thinking, as if she knew what I had told my oncologist only hours earlier.

The card read, "From both of us, Mother, The memories we make—the laughter we share—These moments mean more when our mother is there." It seems Isabelle wants me to fight harder and for me to be here for as long as I possibly can. I just don't know if I can do that . . .

27

Dreams Reborn

Nothing says "commitment to living" quite like taking out a mortgage. At the beginning of summer 2015, Josh and I had some very exciting news. And no, unfortunately, it was not the shocking discovery that the scans showing mets in my lungs were in fact someone else's—I wish. The news was that Josh and I signed a contract to purchase the apartment next door for the purpose of combining it with our current apartment to create a 2,529-square-foot abode that will likely feature four and a half bedrooms (two of which will be master bedrooms) and three and a half baths. For those of you who are not aware of the nature of New York City real estate, the opportunity to purchase a neighboring apartment and create a proper living space is a rare occurrence. That opportunity is even more unique in a well-constructed and landmarked building, as is the case here. The influx of money from foreign investors who find New York real estate to be a safer depository for their wealth than their home countries' banking systems has driven real estate prices to levels that are unfathomable to those who do not live in this city. It has also pushed purchasers out of Manhattan and into the less expensive surrounding boroughs, particularly Brooklyn (which is where we live).

Already feeling the need for more space with two little girls, Josh and I were daydreaming about the possibility of buying a neighbor's apartment right around the time I was diagnosed, as unlikely as that was (although I had not asked Josh to lay precise odds on just how unlikely). But what was improbable two years ago has come to pass—our neighbors have outgrown their apartment and are selling their two-bedroom home to us.

Even though I had had this on my mind for more than two years, when I learned that the neighbors were going to sell their place, the thought of purchasing the apartment didn't cross my mind. Instead, I thought, Oh no, Mia and Belle will lose another playmate in the building. I didn't even think to say anything to Josh for an entire week. But when I did tell him, "H and T are selling and moving," Josh's eyes opened wide, and he asked excitedly, "Are you serious? This is our chance!" I looked at him blankly, not understanding what he was saying.

There is a condition known as chemo brain. Any patient who has been subjected to prolonged infusions of chemotherapy knows it well. Chalk my momentary incomprehension up to that.

In the time it took for me to understand what Josh was saying, and before I could allow myself to envision a gloriously expanded apartment, all the horrible complications that cancer might bring to bear on an ambitious construction project like this flashed through my mind. As much as I can push cancer to the recesses of my consciousness, especially when I'm on vacation or otherwise truly living in the moment, any action or consideration that requires even the slightest contemplation of the future is always burdened by the movements and behavior of my cancer and its impact on my mind and body.

What if in the middle of renovations, I needed surgery and could not oversee the project (because it would be me, and not Josh, who would be wearing the hard hat). What if, worse yet, I died before the new apartment was done? How would Josh, who is so atrocious about the finer details of life, manage? What if we had to move out of our apartment? What about the financial obligations, and what if we needed the money for some surgery or other treatment not covered by insurance? What if . . . what if . . . *what if* . . .

I instantly also saw the wonderful potential of what Josh was pro-
posing—a phenomenal investment, an apartment where the girls
would have their own rooms (because I was sure at some point they
would tire of sharing their full-size bed), a place big enough to accommodate my parents and in-laws and others who can and will help me,
Josh, and the girls as I become sicker and after I die, a place big enough
to accommodate a hospice bed when the time comes (as I had often
wondered whether I would be able to spend my last days in this home
that I love given the space constraints). Four-bedroom apartments
with that kind of square footage are highly coveted commodities in
New York City, and if constructed well, ours would be a wonderful
place in which the girls would grow and thrive, a place that could be
passed down from generation to generation, a labor of love by me, and
the single greatest physical and tangible legacy I could leave for my
children and husband. For both Josh and me, it would represent the
realization of an ambitious dream that harkens back to the precancer
days and, despite the cancer, evidence that life can and does go on after
an appalling diagnosis, even an incurable one; it would be a powerful
symbolic affirmation of life and living and optimism for a future that is
bigger than me.

But what about all the what-ifs? My mind went into problem-
solving mode. We consulted with our financial advisers and pored over
detailed cash-flow analyses. We spoke to architects, bankers, lawyers,
Realtors, building representatives, and others. Based on those many
conversations, we grew comfortable that a combination was doable
from every perspective, including design and construction, legality,
and financing (including the assurance that we would not need to
move out of our current apartment since nearly all of the work would
be done in the other apartment and would be completed before any
walls were torn down between the two units).

But with respect to my paramount concern—that the cancer might
rob me of the ability to oversee this project—I spoke to my brother
and sister. They both instantly loved the idea; among all the obvious
benefits, they believed that a project like this would keep me going.
More practically, my sister is an architect by training, and I knew, and

she confirmed, that if I were not able to complete the oversight of this project, she would be ready, willing, and able to step in. Of course, so much of the decision making would come initially, during the design and planning phase (especially when the right professionals were hired), and I have every intention of being around to set the plans in place. And then it will just be a matter of those professionals executing based on the plans.

As my sister told me, the most important person in this whole process would be the contractor and, fortunately for me, I have a contractor whom I absolutely adore. Now, how often do you hear that statement? He worked on the redesign of our living room last December, the month when I learned of my recurrence and incurable status. The poor guy chose the wrong time to call me, days after I received the news, and ask me how I was doing, for which he got an earful of my tears. I think he must feel really sorry for me, because since then he's been so very kind and concerned and has even come by to replace lightbulbs. What contractor makes house calls after finishing his job to change lightbulbs?

I asked him to come by a couple weekends ago to look at the other apartment so he could give me a very preliminary cost estimate, during which I had a frank discussion with him about how I would need to be able to trust him to carry out my wishes if I got too ill or did not survive long enough to see this through to the end. He was immediately alarmed, wanting to know if there had been negative health developments. I assured him that I was stable for the moment, but I had to always prepare for the worst. He looked me in the eye, put his hand on my shoulder, and declared, "Nothing is going to happen to you. I'm not going to let anything happen to you." I was so moved by his obvious concern and his belief that he could somehow affect the course of my disease. That kind of support is priceless.

Ever since I was diagnosed, I've learned that so much of life's hardship becomes more bearable when you are able to build and lean on a network of loyalty, support, and love, and gather around you people (even your contractor) who will stand by you and help you. But the thing is you have to let them in; you have to let them see the heartache,

pain, and vulnerability, and not cloak those things in a shameful darkness, and then you have to let those people who care about you help
you.

Finally, I asked my oncologist for his blessing. I felt like I needed this
most of all; actually, his blessing was the only one that truly mattered
to me. Not that he could see the future, exactly, but he knew more
about what was inside of me than anyone. His response was rather
comical in its briefness in light of how much thought I had given to the
cancer in making this decision. "Do it!" he said. Brevity really is the
soul of wit. My cancer, this thing that has often felt like it controls
every part of me and my life, seemed to be such a nonissue to him in
this regard.

And with Dr. A.C.'s blessing, we moved forward. It would be a few
months before we could start the construction work, since we still had
to decide on the conceptual designs, obtain building and city approv-
als, and finalize the financing. But signing the contract was the first big
step.

It took me two solid years of living with metastatic cancer to realize an important truth: barring some physical pain or other impedi-
ment brought on by cancer or its treatment, it isn't cancer that denies
me my dreams; it isn't cancer that would prevent me from going on
vacations or buying a new home or doing anything else that I long to
do. Rather, it is a paralyzed mind succumbing to the fear and unpre-
dictability of cancer that would deny me my dreams. In its paralysis, it
groups into one category all dreams that are truly gone (such as having
another biological child) with dreams that can be reshaped and rede-
fined, or even new dreams that are derivative of a cancer diagnosis. In
its paralysis, the mind cannot form contingency plans; it cannot be
brave and bold and forward thinking; it cannot accept what *is* without
running from *what will be*.

In one of the many ironies that have come with having an incurable
prognosis, it is as if by accepting the inevitability of my death from this
disease, I have freed myself from that paralysis. Similarly, I can move
forward now with some degree of certainty; I can plan for myself and
my family, for as much as I emphasize living in the here and now, living
and loving those whom we love by necessity requires some degree of

planning, of thinking about what might be, of dreaming for them if not necessarily for ourselves.

I rejoice in my liberation, in my own courage to move forward, in the rebirth of a dream I once thought was forever lost to me.

Live while you live, my friends.

28

Solitude

I am being brutally honest, as part of my commitment to give voice to all those I know who feel as I do, and to depict the dark side of cancer and debunk the overly sweet, pink-ribbon façade of positivity and fanciful hope and rah-rah-rah nonsense spewed by cancer patients and others, which I have come to absolutely loathe. I believe, as I have always believed, that in honesty—a brutal yet kind and thoughtful honesty—we ultimately find not vulnerability, shame, and disgrace, but liberation, healing, and wholeness. I hope my family and friends do not take offense at this honesty.

In early August 2015, I received some bad scan results, which made for a somewhat difficult couple of weeks. Because bad news seems to come in multiples, a few days later, I learned that my ever-so-historically-reliable tumor marker (CEA) had risen yet again, another 7 points to 29, the largest single increase in a three-week period yet. For me, clicking on that link that reveals the latest CEA results is more stressful than hearing my scan results, probably because my CEA has always told me what to expect in the scans. For those of you who don't know what it's like to find out what your CEA is when you have metastatic cancer and the result is not good, it's like having my heart collapse into my stomach; the walls close in and I feel a primal panic and desperation I imagine an animal pursued by a predator must feel as it realizes it's caught.

Curled up in a fetal position on my bed was how my children found me after I had clicked on the CEA link. Belle asked me why I was crying. "Mommy is just really sad," I told her. My sweet and uniquely perceptive girl then gave me a hug and declared, "Don't worry, Mommy. I'm still going to love you when I grow up." You see, I do fear that in my absence, my children's memories of me will fade and they will love me less and less over time. Her words made me weep with a renewed vigor. Josh came home shortly thereafter. I told him about the CEA results and cried into his neck. He acted so calm and strong for me even though I knew he was upset. Even so, sometimes I think the intensity and ferocity of my emotions are too much for him, especially since he has to come to terms with his own. He urged me to call my sister or my best friend, anyone. The only person I wanted to talk to was my therapist, but she was away until September. Usually, as expressive as I am in writing, I have the same compunction to verbally unload my heartaches to those closest to me in life (besides Josh), because I know that for me the process of verbalization is healing. But not now. I didn't and still don't even want to talk to people who have my disease, at least not anyone who is in a better position than I am, and I imagine anyone who is in a worse position doesn't want to talk to me. My self-imposed reclusiveness and isolationism is partly because of the jealousy and the hate.

I cannot imagine anyone saying anything to me that would be remotely helpful or comforting. I don't want to hear about the promise of immunotherapy. I don't want words of sympathy. I don't want sage words of advice about how to live the remainder of my life. I don't want to talk about it. I don't want to answer any questions. I don't want to have to be forced to explain anything to anyone. Whatever explanations I give and whatever information I divulge must be on my terms and at my initiation, not because someone asked or because I was forced into some social interaction.

Perhaps isolation, at least emotionally if not physically, is what happens as you get closer to death, as you understand more powerfully than ever before that this journey to the end is one that must be made absolutely alone. It feels as if whatever comfort there is will be found within, rather than without, from private conversations with my innermost self and, when I can muster belief, the gods.

I heard back from the surgeon in Germany about the laser surgery. I now have too many mets in my lungs, forty in each one, and too many are centrally located. I am inoperable. This laser surgery is supposed to be able to resect up to one hundred mets in each lung. It was sickening to hear that I'm not even a candidate for it, more sickening than hearing about yet another CEA rise. The other surgeon, in the United Kingdom, never got back to me. I see no point in pursuing him further since he's a student of the German surgeon, and I can't imagine his opinion will be any different. I suppose that's 24,000 euros saved and I won't have to spend weeks away from my children. That's what I told myself, anyway, to make myself feel better.

I've been crying a lot, in bed, at the gym, during acupuncture, in restaurants. It's not as bad as it was in those dark days of December and January. I'm still engaging the world. I acted relatively normal at Belle's fourth birthday party. I have even managed to see a couple friends. I still laugh and think a lot about other things besides cancer.

The night after I heard from the German surgeon, I was lying in bed between Mia and Isabelle. Belle had fallen asleep, but Mia was still awake and demanding that I tell her a story. I like to tell her stories about my life and my family growing up. She loves to hear about my and my family's escape from Vietnam, but that night, in my heightened emotional state, I wanted to tell her another story about me, something she'd never heard before. I had been talking to her about the virtues of discipline and hard work as they pertained to her violin practice. Even though she's been studying violin for only three months, her teacher has repeatedly told me and Josh that Mia is exceptionally talented. She seems to have inherited Josh's incredible musical ability.

Not long after her lessons began, I was sitting in on one of them and was so impressed by the sounds coming out of her instrument. I said to the teacher, "You know, I'm really glad I decided to rent such a high-quality violin for Mia. It sounds really good." Her teacher responded, "Actually, I've had plenty of students who have played on expensive violins and they did not sound good. Mia is really talented." I was shocked. It had never occurred to me that my daughter could actually be gifted at the violin. Of course, I *would* think that the nice sounds coming out of the instrument were because of the instrument, not because of my daughter! It was such a Chinese mom moment, so deprecating, so doubtful. My mother said things like that about me and my siblings all the time. If you're Chinese, you will understand.

Ever since then, I've made a conscious effort to really believe in and nurture Mia's musical ability to make up for my Chinese mom moment (and to resist the voice of skepticism when it tells me that the teacher is exaggerating). So I've been pushing her to practice daily, which is like pulling teeth without novocaine at times. Recently, rather than rewarding her with stickers and toys for practicing, I've been trying to explain to her that the goal (among others) is to instill in her a sense of discipline, although I'm not sure how much a five-year-old understands or cares about the virtue of discipline and its implications for life. So that night, I thought I would make the point through one of my stories.

I gathered Mia close, and we lay on our sides like a couple of nesting spoons, her long, spindly arms and legs tucked in as tight as possible and the bright hallway light casting a reassuring glow on the wall at which we were staring. And I began:

Mommy is going to tell you a story about Mommy that you haven't really heard before. You know Mommy was born in Vietnam, but did you know I was blind when I was born? It was after the war, and there was no food or money, no money for Neh and Gong [what Mia calls my parents] to pay a doctor to make Mommy better. And even if they did have the money, there were no doctors in Vietnam that would have known how to fix Mommy's eyes. But somehow we found a way out, and eventually we made it to this country, the United States. And even though we didn't have any money, because nice people gave us money, Mommy was able to go to one of the best eye doctors in the world, and he fixed Mommy's eyes. But even he couldn't make them perfect. I still can't see very well. That's why I always ask you to help me see. You are my eyes sometimes.

I was really sad a lot when I was little because I couldn't see like

Uncle or Titi or Mommy's cousins. I wanted to be able to ride a bike and play tennis and drive a car. I wanted not to have to use big books with superbig words. And no one understood how Mommy felt. I was alone and sometimes lonely in my world of half-blindness. Because Mommy couldn't see very well, everyone in Mommy's family thought I was not very smart. They didn't think Mommy could do anything. Mommy got really mad. I didn't like people telling me what I could or couldn't do, and I was determined to show them that I could do anything I wanted. Remember that, Mia: only you can determine for yourself what you are capable of; no one else can, not even Mommy or Daddy.

So Mommy worked really, *really* hard and exercised a lot of discipline. I studied a lot, and then people started to realize that even though I couldn't see well, that didn't mean I was dumb or that I couldn't do anything with my life. I got really good grades in school and ended up going to a good college. I traveled all over the world by myself, which isn't easy when you can't see well. I found a good job. And do you know what was the best part, Mia? Finding Daddy and then having you and Belle. I never thought I would be able to find someone like your daddy who would love me so much, and neither did anyone else, it seemed, and all because I couldn't see like everybody else. I never thought I could get married and have kids. I never thought anyone would want me. You, Belle, and Daddy are the best things that ever happened to me. But everything good in my life started because I was willing to work hard, to be determined and disciplined because I wanted something for myself so very much. That's why I want you to learn the value of working hard. Don't ever forget this story, okay? I want you to remember Mommy's story forever.

Mia was quiet for a minute, and I knew she was processing in her quick brain what I had just told her. Then she said, "I won't forget, Mommy, but you should write it down. Then when I'm bigger and I can read better, I can read the story and remind myself."

29

A Game of Clue

Lately my thoughts have been trapped inside an exhausted mind.

I've been busy thinking about bathroom tiles and flooring and gilded wallpaper, calculating costs and pondering the finer details of the proposed layout. How I wish that my life was made up entirely of mundaneness, for I am so sick of existentialism. But alas, simplicity and normalcy have never been and will never be my destiny.

The cancer part of my life has dominated of late. In early September, I sank into the darkness of a new abyss, one characterized by anger, bitterness, hate, and paralyzing loneliness. The recent loss of two true friends, combined with the horrible side effects from my most recent treatment plan, has pushed me over the edge.

These were friends whom I saw from time to time, and whom I visited a few weeks before they died. Chris was a kind soul, beloved husband, father, brother, son, and friend, chess player and teacher and, least of all, my mentor of sorts on this cancer journey. He listened to my ramblings over lunch or tea, observed how I had grown over the months from the belligerent warrior who was determined to beat this cancer to the more contemplative philosopher who seeks above all else to find meaning, peace, and acceptance in a life over which I have little control. Cancer, at least for me, truly is a journey that makes me question and analyze all my beliefs about myself (as in whether I am strong or weak, brave or cowardly), about the existence of a higher being and its role in the affairs of mankind, about commitment and love (as in how far will I go to stay alive for my family), about the meaning of my life and life in general, about death and what awaits.

If you are open to these inevitable questions, which only something like incurable cancer can force into the forefront of your mind, if you allow yourself the time and patience to mull over these complex, baffling, painful, and impossible queries, the journey will both change you (for the better, I believe) and make you more of who you have always been.

Chris understood that long before I did. We shared a similar philosophy, heavily influenced by Buddhist thought, but he was wiser than I, and so he was a teacher to me. I went to see him as he was entering hospice care. We sat on his terrace with a view of the Atlantic Ocean and talked of his sadness and expectations, and I marveled at his genuine lack of bitterness, anger, and fear; he was grace and dignity personified. As I said my final farewell, knowing that I would never see him again, I hugged him and asked him to wait for me on the other side. He said he would, and that gives me great comfort.

Chris was the first true friend I lost to colon cancer. Yes, I've written about others, but they were more in the nature of virtual friends. I didn't meet them for lunch. I didn't visit them in their homes.

J was another friend I would see from time to time, most often in her Manhattan apartment, which spoke of a fruitful life. I never knew just how famous J was until I saw her obituary in *The New York Times*. You have to be someone relatively important to have your obituary written by a third party and published in *The New York Times,* no less. But J always downplayed her professional success—she was a renowned animator with forty years of prolific work behind her, work that has been displayed at MoMA and the Met for its innovative significance—and I had absolutely no idea. To each other, we were simply two women, two wives, two mothers, suffering from the same horrible disease. We met to discuss the pros and cons of HIPEC surgery. She was an extremely private person when it came to her cancer, and so I was perhaps the only person in the cancer community she befriended and spoke to on a somewhat regular basis, and one of the few friends she allowed into her clouded world. She gave my children two books she had written and illustrated and an app on the iPad to help them learn the alphabet. I was shocked by her death, for it happened too quickly for me. At our last meeting, just before the summer, she didn't look like she was going to die so soon. In fact, I told her in an email that her desire to go into hospice seemed premature; she never replied. I would learn subsequently that she died two weeks later, at the end of June, with a disease progression that astounded even her doctors. I didn't get a chance to say a proper goodbye, which I regret deeply.

I regret it because she was my friend, but I also regret it because although most normal people are scared to be around dying people, I find that other dying people are not scared. I am not scared. Because J just arrived at my ultimate destination. She was simply on an earlier train, is all. That proximity to death is a powerful draw to a dying person—to be near it, to commune with it, to give and take comfort from it.

Apart from the departure of friends, which can never be mastered, I feel that I have just about otherwise mastered the rhythms of this elaborate game of Clue known as Stage IV disease: You fall in and out of love with doctors. You may even be tempted to cheat on your oncologist, have flings with other major hospitals, only to go back home to your faithful oncologist with your tail between your legs. You will enthusiastically embrace different modalities, only to see them collapse. Different drug combinations or clinical trials will have you convinced that each of them is the *one*. It is not the one. You will spend time and money on alternative therapies, only to be alternately frustrated and *really* frustrated. You will, throughout, be a basket case, and you will scream and cry and then you will wipe your face and meet with plumbers and look at samples for the new master bedroom that you're in charge of, then go have dinner with friends. Because life must be lived!

Nearly two months ago, after the surgeon in Germany told me laser surgery on my lungs was not possible, I made the decision, with the support of my oncologist, to start the drug Erbitux (generically known as the even harder to pronounce cetuximab). Erbitux is the drug for which Martha Stewart gave up a few months of her freedom. It is an option only for patients who do not have the KRAS mutation in their tumors, for in patients with that mutation, it seems to do more harm than good. So I suppose I am lucky to be KRAS wild (i.e., normal), since that mutation is actually quite common, affecting 40 to 60 percent of the colorectal cancer population. Erbitux comes with nasty side effects, including bad rashes and acne. However, because it is a targeted therapy, it tends to be gentle on the blood counts and platelets.

I told Dr. A.C. in no uncertain terms, "I want to die from the cancer, not from the treatment for the cancer."

He responded, "How about you not die at all?" His unexpectedly optimistic question brought a wary smile to my heart. Only from him can I tolerate such syrupy optimism. No one else. His comment was so contrary to the dim prognosis he had given me last December that I must believe all this immunotherapy buzz that has gained such ferocity in the interim has actually given him a real sense of possibility. And when he believes, I can muster the courage to believe, too, just a little.

I went on to inform Dr. A.C. unequivocally, "I don't want my children to remember me so sick." He responded, "In this case, they'll just remember you with acne."

I would also be going back on a maintenance course of the chemo drug 5-FU, administered every two weeks over a forty-eight-hour period through a pump that one must carry around. I did not want to wear the pump, in part because it's annoying but mostly because my children and Josh get upset when they see this obvious sign of my illness. Dr. A.C. then proposed something I'd never heard of (at least not in today's standard of care); since I would be receiving the Erbitux on a weekly basis, he could give me a quick injection of the 5-FU at each infusion as well. That seemed like the perfect solution. I agreed.

I had made my treatment decisions, and I felt good about them. I'm fortunate in having an oncologist who listens to me and allows me to make my own treatment decisions, as frightening as that can be. He is willing to do what is unusual, to try the unorthodox. As he has said, "Just because it's not typically done doesn't mean we can't do it." And most of all, I love the fact that we follow each other on Instagram, that we allow each other to see other personal parts of our lives, that we talk about our gardening endeavors and our children. I think that the relationship between a patient with metastatic cancer and his or her oncologist should be a special one, unlike any other patient-doctor relationship. Because oncology is all about where life meets death, the relationship should go beyond the medicine and the science; it should be about our mutual humanity. I need to feel that bond with the doctor who will either save my life or, much more likely, walk with me toward the end of my life.

But whatever goodness I felt about my treatment decisions was short-lived. Within a week, my face had developed the expected rash and acne, what my dermatologist called pustules. It's a disgusting word, yet it so aptly described what was happening on my face. Clindamycin (a topical cream) and doxycycline (an oral antibiotic) quickly brought the rash and acne under control (although my face still looks flushed all the time). My scalp started to itch and grew sore to the touch, a general precursor to hair loss. Sure enough, I started losing hair a few weeks ago. I've begun using hair masques to promote more moisture to my scalp and hair in the hope that doing so will mitigate the hair loss.

About a week after my first Erbitux infusion, I developed a floater in my left eye. Everyone gets floaters from time to time, but because of my previous eye surgeries, I'm more prone to them. My previous floaters would always go away after a few days, but this one didn't. They've always been disconcerting to me because they bring to mind the possibility of worsening eyesight and blindness, which for someone with my history is among the greatest of fears. When I was little, I used to call them flies dancing around my field of vision; I had no other way to tell my mother about the dark spot that was there no matter where I looked and even when I closed my eyes.

I also developed a strange, tender lump near the base of my neck, which Dr. A.C. doesn't think is a brain met, unless my brain has grown out of my skull, but we have no idea what it is. For now, we simply watch it as I push it around with my fingers. I draw little comfort from the fact that my recent brain MRI showed nothing.

But such vain concerns as acne and hair loss, annoying eye floaters and bizarre lumps on my head, and even the frequent fatigue pale in comparison to the skin breaks on my hands, feet, and lips from the extreme dryness and the mouth sores. Despite frequent applications of lotions and creams, I would wake up with dried blood caked on my lips and in the beds of my fingernails. However, the mouth sores win, hands down. They are the worst side effect I have experienced since being in treatment. Worse than any nausea, constipation, diarrhea, neuropathy, anything! And that is what my medical team has been truly concerned about, for mouth sores can reduce appetite and inhibit eating and the all-important intake of critical nutrients. The existing mouthwashes and remedies to address the mouth sores have been generally ineffective. A new sore would appear on my tongue, gums, or the insides of my lips and cheeks just as one was about to go away. One sore at the back of my tongue caused burning pain in my ear canal every time I ate. I was outraged at the absurdity of mouth pain traveling into my ears! I mean, cancer can kill you, but must it also play such games?

At one point I could barely speak because moving my mouth to talk was too painful, and I told the girls I could not read them bedtime stories. Water is barely tolerable. Eating has generally become a tortured and slow process, as there is stinging everywhere in my mouth when food enters (although I have to admit the coolness and creaminess of ice cream really soothes the raging fire). For someone who loves to cook (and eat) as much as I do, the pain in my mouth has truly been excruciating and borderline intolerable. At my doctor's insistence and with my happy acquiescence, I skipped treatment over Labor Day week to give my mouth and fingers more time to heal.

I have been reminded how pain can sap your spirit and destroy your will. Perhaps, to my shame, I just don't have a very high pain tolerance. Sadly, that's not something I can change. Pain makes me miserable, as it does everyone. But this physical pain, the emotional pain I was already in, exacerbated by the deaths of my friends, and the stresses of having to deal with the other side effects, drove me into the darkest of abysses.

On a Sunday night, on the eve of yet another treatment and with my mouth on fire, I couldn't get Isabelle to go to bed and I lost my shit, as they say. I yelled and screamed at her. Josh told me I had crossed the line. I sat on the couch and cried because of the terrible mother I was becoming, because the pain and misery of everything was turning me into a mother and wife I didn't want to be. I cried into the wee hours of the night, sitting alone in the dark. Never in my life have I cried with such intensity and despair. Never have I felt so weakened and alone. I seriously considered stopping treatment because I didn't want my children to remember me this way. Desperate for help, I posted this on the Colon Club forum:

> For quite a while now, ever since I last posted about my sense of loneliness and solitude, I haven't reached out to anyone to talk about what's going on . . . I've convinced myself that nothing anyone can say can comfort me. I'm filled with so much jealousy, bitterness, and hate, I don't know what to do to let those feelings go. For months I thought I had found peace, but then the most recent scan results came, and my brief period of stability is over. I don't feel like my husband can understand, nor my friends. The only people who can understand are those who are in my exact position, but no such person exists.
>
> But tonight, I logged in here after a long absence, looking for some relief. Desperate, I suppose. The Erbitux I've been on now for a month is causing my mouth such discomfort. It's miserable. The rash I can manage, so I won't even complain about that. I'm also convinced Erbitux has caused this persistent floater in my left eye, which makes me want to rip the eye out of my head. If you know my history of vision issues (blindness at birth, blah, blah, blah), then maybe you'll

understand how this would aggravate me and creates anxiety about whether Erbitux might cause blindness or something. Anyhow, tonight I lost my shit with my four-year-old daughter, who refused to go to bed. I know it was a reaction to all this cancer crap. I don't want to live like this. I don't want my children to remember me as a bitch in pain and unhappy. I have my next treatment tomorrow, and I told my husband I want to stop. I would rather die sooner than live like this. I'd rather feel good and be happy and be a good mother. I know I don't have the courage to actually follow through with that statement, but in time I will.

We recently started going to church because Mia insisted. I'm not a Christian and I never will be, but I go to church to support my husband (who was raised an Episcopalian) and children. I politely refuse communion in lieu of the blessing, but I do listen to the sermon with as open a mind as I can. One sermon in particular by Mother Kate has stayed with me. She spoke of how while we often emphasize the power and goodness of the light, sometimes wonderful things can come out of darkness, too. She held up a plant from her Brooklyn apartment, which, like so many other apartments in the city, is in short supply of natural light. She spoke of how it started as a seed in the dark depth of the soil. This is also true of all human and animal life; we all begin in the dark, do we not?

On that night, I cried and I cried. In what seemed like a symbolic gesture of how low I had gone, I dropped to the floor and cried on the rug, sobbing inconsolably into the pile. And then, in that lonely darkness, my precious Isabelle, the same child I had raged at only hours before, came to me. She found me on the rug and, for many minutes, she sat next to me, putting her hand on my head and saying nothing, as I continued to weep.

Then she asked in her sweet little four-year-old voice, "Mommy, why are you lying on the floor?"

The more metaphorical answer was of course impossible for me to say to her, so I gave her a simple answer: "Because Mommy is hot."

A comfortable silence fell between us. Then, I said, "Isabelle, you should go back to your bed and go to sleep."

Her response: "But, Mommy, I want you to come sleep with me. You can sleep on the floor in my room, if you want."

How could I refuse this child of mine who had ventured into the darkness to extend her hand and offer love and forgiveness to her awful mother? I slept between her and Mia on their full-size bed the rest of the night, shunning the floor.

30

The Gift of Grief

The most frequent question I get, after "How are you?," is "How are the girls doing?"

My children are very aware that I am sick, that I will likely die before too much more time has passed. Slowly, as they have grown older, they have understood more and more what "death" means, although of course I doubt they have a true understanding of what my death would mean to them emotionally.

My so-smart, almost six-year-old Mia quietly tries to intellectualize all of this, break it down to its component parts, and analyze it. She likes to watch documentaries about wild animals killing each other. She loves to sit on her daddy's lap and watch shows about airplane crashes in which death is reenacted and then the investigators come in to solve the mystery of why the plane fell out of the sky. She watches forensic autopsy shows about gruesome murders and how science is used to find the murderers. Josh finds such morbid shows captivating, and apparently so does his elder daughter, since she watches them with exceptional focus. Other than the wildlife shows, every time Mia and Josh turn such shows on, Belle protests, screaming, "I don't *wanna* watch airplane crash shows!" and runs into another room, frequently dragging me with her.

It was on one such occasion, while father and daughter were watching a show and Josh was explaining to Mia the meaning of "A.D." as in the year A.D. 1532 and its association with the crucifixion of Jesus, that Mia expressed her desire to go to church, to learn more about Jesus, and said that she believed herself to be a Christian. Since we don't talk to her much about religion (and indeed Mia had never before been to church), I'm sure she has been having conversations about God and religion at school, likely with one of her classmates who goes to church. But Mia has been speaking of God since she was four, so it wasn't all that surprising to me when she expressed this desire to learn more about Christianity. I remember a couple of occasions when we would walk by a church soon after I was diagnosed and she would ask me, "What is that building?" or "Who made us, Mommy?"

And then there are the infrequent conversations between her and Belle as they lie in bed:

Belle: God is dead.

Mia: No, he's not. He's everywhere. He made us.

So that is why we have started going to church and embracing the community it represents. And I go too, even though I am not Christian, because I want to encourage my family to avail themselves of whatever they can to help them through trying times. I trust that my children are intelligent and discerning and will determine for themselves at a later time, when they have greater maturity and knowledge, whether Christianity or some other religion or belief, if any, is appropriate for them.

Belle, however, does not seem so into the church thing. She likes Sunday school, now that it has restarted, but sitting through the services, however short and catered to children they may be, can be challenging for her.

This was the conversation we had as we were walking to church one day:

Belle (whining): Mommy, why do we have to go to church every day?

Me: We don't go to church every day. We go only on Sundays.

Belle (defiantly): Friday is my favorite day because on Fridays, I get to eat pizza and I don't have to go to church!

Even as Isabelle wishes for me to live, I know she is preparing for my death. I think preparation is a good thing, a very good thing for both of my children. I think it will ease the pain and the grief, but more important, it allows them to process that horrible scenario while I'm still here, so I can help them through it; so they can unleash their anger or whatever emotion at me or the world, and then I can soothe them; so they can ask me questions, as they have been doing; so they know from me directly how much I love them and will always love them.

I think of this as the "gift of grief." We grieve together, now, and weep for their loss and for my passing, now, so that they are not left to figure it out on their own after I have suddenly vanished. Some mental health professionals recommend sparing small children this part of the dying process, but in my view and for my children, heeding that advice would mean sparing them a level of feeling and affection that is unparalleled, a mother love that will make lasting memories, and that they may never know again in their lives.

Isabelle once asked Josh when they were sitting in the car together, "Can I sit in Mommy's seat after she dies?" And then one night at bedtime, she wanted to tell the stories, instead of me telling the stories. So she told two stories, with completely contrary themes. The first story was about salvation (possibly mine): "Once upon a time there was a dragon and a princess. The dragon ate the princess. The prince cut a hole in the dragon's stomach, went inside, and took the princess out. Then, they lived happily ever after."

And then she told her second story: "Once upon a time there was a frog and a princess. The frog ate the princess. And then the prince found a new princess and they lived happily ever after. The end."

Isabelle's behavior is so often uncanny. She exhibits an ageless soul that astounds me time and time again. In the moments when I believe in a God, I feel the power of this child of mine, and I am convinced that she was brought to me to help me deal with my disease. Or perhaps, more accurately, it is when I witness this child's wisdom, her singular understanding of me, her magic, that I believe in a God, even that God speaks to me through her.

When Mia hugs me with her long limbs, I feel her love; I feel her need for me to bolster her being and her need for me to assure her that I love her no less than I love her sister. I wish I could explain to her the incredible grace, beauty, intelligence, and kindness that I already see in her despite her tender age, and I marvel with pride that I produced such a lovely, lovely being. Indeed, I love both of them without end and marvel constantly at how I could be a mother to these amazing girls. I feel a love for them I never knew possible.

But Belle's hugs are different. When Isabelle hugs me with her more compact, stockier body (for she is all solid torso and meaty flesh, while her willowy sister is all impossibly long legs and arms), I feel her love, yes, but there is not the same neediness from her. Rather, I feel like the weight of her body holds me to this earth and to this life in those moments when I want to leave it most, as if in her embrace she is silently telling me that I must live not for her but because there is more for my soul to do and learn in this life, that I have more to give to the world before I move on, that my presence in this life has served and continues to serve a greater good than just taking care of her and her sister.

So now with all of that said, you will understand what it meant to me for Isabelle to come into my darkness that lonely, miserable night and bring me out, to extend her hand to lift me off the floor of my abyss.

I woke up the next morning, exhausted but clear-eyed and resolute. I knew that I and my family had grown tired and bored of the narrative of self-pity I had constructed for myself over the previous weeks and months. I knew that I had to do something to pull myself out of my darkness. Isabelle had offered her hand, but I had to do the remainder of the work.

2016

31

In Which the Yips Come to America

I am sitting on my grandmother's lap. I can feel the rocking of the boat—right now the rocking is gentle, but I know it is not always so. I can see the eerie glow of a bare incandescent bulb dangling from somewhere above and a cloudy night sky that is not completely black. I can hear the motor. *Chuk . . . chuk . . . chuk.* But most of all, I hear the strident voices of the people around me—there are so many people—human voices of desperation that are louder than those of the boat and the ocean. I can tell that the people are talking skyward, to something or someone in the night sky. I understand their words. They say things like "Please, God, please help us," and "Dear God, please look after us." And there, with my head lying on my grandmother's chest, I, too, look toward the sky, staring at its gray-blackness, and I think for a second that I hear a voice from the clouds. But then, I think it was just my own longing to hear an answer to the prayers, because I understand instinctively that what these people are praying for is important to all of us. I understand that their prayers are about wanting to live and not die, and I want to live, too.

Then I feel the hunger gnawing at my stomach again, and I cry out for more milk, banging my empty bottle against my grandmother's lap, fighting for food in the only way I know how, in the only way I can. My grandmother yells at me. She is angry with me.

"There is no more milk! Do you hear me? And there won't be any milk anytime soon no matter how much you cry. So shut up!" She snatches my baby bottle from me and hurls it, spinning, into the black sea, as if doing so will make everything better. A part of me knows that she would have liked to throw me overboard instead, but she can't.

I cry even harder. I can't stop crying.

It is on the boat that my first real and conscious memories of the world were formed. I say real and conscious because these images and sensations are the first memories in which I recall something more than just vague flashes of color and light, the first memories that have always floated more in the realm of reality than dream, remembered by my mind and not just my soul, and the first memories in which I have comprehension of the world around me and a self-awareness of my own existence within that world. Nascent though that comprehension might have been, I grasped the desperation of the moment and the precariousness of my own life. On that boat, I learned fear, hunger, and the desire to live.

The boat was such a primal and frightening experience that afterward it would cause most members of my family to try to rid the experience from their consciousness, never to speak of it again. It was so primal and frightening that the memories of it still make my mother shudder every time she sees an endless expanse of ocean, prompting her to declare even after so many years, "I would have never dared to get on that boat had I known . . ." But, of course, she didn't know, and therefore she dared.

That we are even here to testify to our flight from Vietnam, that we survived, beggars belief. Before we had even embarked, the water, already a foot deep in the ship's hold, poured in through its battered hull, and the boat settled more and more deeply into the water. People rushing to find a place to settle down on the open boat's one and only deck could see the water when they scurried past the short flight of stairs that led below. Yet none of them seemed to care, for no one tried to get off and more continued to come on board. Apparently they believed, bravely or perhaps stupidly, as my parents and so many others before them believed: Better to die at sea than to live in Vietnam. Better to get on a sinking boat than to stay one more moment on Vietnamese soil.

But then a voice of sanity cut through the drone of the boat's engine and the din of the crowd.

"Get rid of luggage! We have to lighten the boat!" Brother Can yelled to the hundred people or so who had already boarded. And then he yelled at the two hundred people still waiting to board the boat via the thick wooden plank that bridged boat and pier, "Only bring what you *need* on board. Nothing else!" And to the boat's helmsman—the person charged with the responsibility of steering the boat—and his brother, standing helplessly nearby, Brother Can pointed and ordered, "Start pumping out the water now! Now, I said!"

Brother Can stood on the port side of the boat, glaring suspiciously at every person who came on board. He was determined to keep order and to stop the boat from sinking before it had even left. After all, the boat was his. Brother Can was technically a brother to only a handful of the passengers; everyone knew who he was, though, and everyone used the word "Brother" as a title of respect (as is common practice in the Vietnamese language). He was the lead organizer of this expedition, the man who had masterminded the acquisition of this boat, approached my grandfather to register the boat in Tam-Ky, and located the helmsman; he was primarily responsible for recruiting and assembling these 315 refugees. People referred to him as the "Boat's Boss," the captain of the boat, and the captain expected his orders to be obeyed.

Brother Can's four younger brothers, tall, beefy, and intimidating like Brother Can himself, moved to do as Brother Can commanded, prepared to forcefully manhandle the luggage of so many complete strangers. The brothers targeted the largest bags squeezed in among the passengers. "Only essentials can come. Just one bag, and not too big!" Brother Can told people again and again as they tried to slip through with loaded backs and hands, as though they were deaf to his instructions. Most of the people Brother Can had to stop turned around and went back to shore to rearrange the belongings from their multiple pieces of luggage so that everything they really wanted and needed would fit in one bag. Those who tried to push past Brother Can came face-to-face with his many brothers-in-law.

Ignoring the cries of outrage at their callous disregard for people's things and knowing that there was no alternative, Brother Can and his relatives tossed, and forced passengers to toss, dozens upon dozens of bulky canvas and nylon bags, straining at zippers and seams, back onto the pier. The wooden pier jutted out from a sandy white beach nestled in a natural harbor protected from the currents of the South China Sea. Sometimes the fishermen from the nearby village of Ky Ha would use this pier to unload fish. But on this dark evening, it was the repository for refugees' abandoned possessions, personal items that had been chosen from a household and a lifetime to be brought with them as they left their native land—clothes, miniature Buddha statues, trinkets, photographs, books, diaries, and a host of other things that had significance only to those who once owned them. Also in those bags were valuable commodities that could be sold in Hong Kong or anywhere else in the world: gold bars and other gold jewelry well in excess of the two taels that the Cong An (the police) permitted each person to take out of the country; thick and fragrant barks of cinnamon trees grown in the jungles of Vietnam that when ground would produce the finest quality cinnamon in the world; and barks of sandalwood that were valued for their perfuming and medicinal powers and could command significant sums of money.

"Don't take my bag! It's not heavy!" a gray-haired woman shrieked, half in protest, half in plea, at one of Brother Can's men. They stood only a few bodies away from where my mother and I sat, me on her lap and she on the wooden deck. After a futile tug-of-war, Brother Can's man wrestled the bag, which was twice the size of the woman's torso, out of her hands, threw it overboard, and then turned to find his next victim.

My mother leaned more heavily against the one bag she had packed for us, pushing it that much harder against the wall at her back, trying to shield it from the man's reach. My grandmother sat next to us, lean-ing against her own bag and the wall. My mother could see my brother sitting next to my father on the bench that ran along the back of the boat. She could see Grandpa arguing with one of Brother Can's broth-ers. My grandfather had brought along a dozen two-foot-long barks of cinnamon, tied together and stuffed into a woven sack that was sup-posed to protect them. Only after my grandfather reminded the man that he had done his part to make this trip possible did the brother re-lent, allowing my grandfather to keep half of the cinnamon bark and throwing the other half onto the pier.

From her position on the floor, off to Brother Can's right, my mother watched the surreal scene unfold in the dim glow of the two bare bulbs that swung freely from the boat's canopy. It was already nine o'clock, past dusk. The Cong An were forcing many boats carting ethnic Chinese to leave at night, fearing that sightings of refugees in flight would encourage the ethnic Vietnamese in their attempts to flee. And so here we all were, maneuvering about in the dark save for the boat's few weak lights. My mother witnessed the yelling and shouting and arguing and negotiating and pressing together of more and more people everywhere; she looked upon the cast-off shreds of people's lives and life savings hurled into the air to lie helter-skelter on the pier where they would be picked over by scavengers by morning. None of this seemed real, not the people being forced to abandon what little they had left after the Communists had already taken so much—some left with just the clothes on their backs—nor the water threatening to drown this tiny, overcrowded boat that was supposed to take three hundred refugees to Hong Kong, more than a thousand miles of open sea to the northeast.

Maybe because it is now winter, I've been thinking a lot about the ghosts of our migration, and of Tobacco Woman, and Grandfather Spirit. And maybe that in turn is a result of not such good scan results, and more recently my bout of severe diarrhea that led me to feel like death.

In Vietnam, on the road outside our house, a Vietnamese woman sold tobacco every day, squatting on the dirt before a cloth that displayed her wares. The spirit of Tobacco Woman's deceased grandfather would sometimes return, and when he did, she would send word to my paternal grandmother. The Grandfather Spirit would often tell my grandmother what numbers to pick in the local lottery—she was an avid gambler—and she would win. But his spirit also advised on much more serious matters, matters of life and death.

My sister, who is six years older than I, developed cataracts at an early age. I suspect they were present in some nascent form when she was born, but they didn't become evident until she was older, maybe around age four. I of course had much more pronounced and obvious cataracts at birth. In any case, neither of our vision problems could be addressed in Vietnam, with even less hope of successful treatment after the Communists won the war.

People fled the country at the time of the fall of Saigon, in 1975, but those early refugees tended to be the Vietnamese who feared reprisal for having sided with the South Vietnamese regime and the American forces.

By 1978, the ethnic Chinese, robbed of their economic freedom, and others were searching for means of unsanctioned escape. Given the clandestine nature of these escapes, it was often the young, single men and women who dared to brave the voyage on rickety fishing boats to locations like Hong Kong and Macau with the hope of eventually reaching a better place. Everyone dreamed of the United States, but other countries such as France, England, and Australia would also do. My third, fourth, and fifth uncles, my father's younger brothers, were the young ones in our family, so they were the ones who dared.

But it was my mother who was the most daring of all. She asked her brothers-in-law to take my eight-year-old sister with them in the hope that Lyna would arrive in a place where her vision could be treated. We would follow later—perhaps to be reunited, perhaps not. Now that I am a mother I can imagine how difficult it must have been to let go of her firstborn child, to know there was the distinct possibility that she might never see her child again, that her child might die on this journey into an unknowable and unimaginable future she'd only glimpsed in movies and fairy tales. My mother tells me now she wanted me to go with my uncles, too, but I was just two years old and too young to thrust upon someone else.

My sister left. Weeks and months went by with no word from the uncles. Mail back then could take six months or longer to arrive, if it arrived at all. My worried mother went to consult Tobacco Woman's Grandfather Spirit when he appeared. He told her that indeed my sister had arrived in America, that she was safe and that all was well. Weeks later, my mother received a letter and enclosed within was a picture of my sister posing with the glorious Golden Gate Bridge behind her, wearing her new American-bought clothes and sporting new glasses.

I realize that many who hear these stories will still not believe in ghosts, and that is perfectly understandable. While I believe in the existence of ghosts and spirits, I also believe that the souls represented by these ghosts and spirits eventually move on to something else, whether it be into a new life or another dimension in time and space, somewhere the soul has a chance to experience more of this universe and to learn. Ultimately, I believe in the evolution of the soul—that the meaning and purpose of life is to enrich the soul with all the joys and heartaches that this life and other lives can impart, that once the soul has learned as much as it can, with all its wisdom and knowledge it enters what the Buddhists would call Nirvana and what Christians might call Heaven and a closeness and even oneness with God.

Since my diagnosis, I've witnessed so much determination to remain alive at all costs, sometimes with a disturbing, maniacal frenzy. I am confident that it is my unwavering belief in ghosts, spirits, reincarnation, and the evolution of my soul that makes me unafraid of dying. Indeed, it is these convictions that will prevent me from clinging to this life and, in some respects, makes me look forward to death. These beliefs lie at the heart of the enduring, evolved, and thoughtful peace that I seek to find with my own death.

Believe what you need to believe in order to find comfort and peace with the inevitable fate that is common to every living thing on this planet. Death awaits us all; one can choose to run in fear from it or one can face it head-on with thoughtfulness, and from that thoughtfulness peace and serenity.

32

Living

On the first day of spring I had a chest CT scan and an abdominal and pelvic MRI. It had been ten weeks since my PET scan in early January, which was "mixed" in that there was some growth, some stability, and some regressions in the various tumors in my lungs. My oncologist and I had agreed that notwithstanding the growth we would continue with the weekly Erbitux infusion and 5-FU push for the time being, but that we would rescan in six weeks as opposed to the more conventional three months. The February rescans showed essential stability, as compared to the January PET, but what was more alarming to me was that they showed "significant" growth from the October CT and MRI.

The different types of scanning technology offer different pros and cons, which I don't pretend to fully understand. I generally get PETs every six to nine months because they can detect disease in the bones as well as metabolic cancer activity in nonsolid areas (e.g., the peritoneum) and cover a more expansive area, from neck to midthigh. While there is a CT scan connected with a PET, the image quality is inferior to that of an actual CT and MRI. All this is by way of explaining that comparing a CT/MRI to a prior CT/MRI is more accurate than comparing a PET to a CT/MRI. Therefore, the change from October to February was more relevant (and disturbing) to me. February's scans showed a couple new tumors and growth of about one to three millimeters in a few others. The MRI also showed an enlarged lymph node in my retroperitoneum that could be cancerous or benign inflammation—radiologists couldn't seem to agree on which. As I had suspected, the Erbitux and 5-FU were starting to fail, if not already completely failing. My oncologist and I agreed, however, that we would hold off on changing treatment until I returned from an upcoming vacation, after which I would rescan and we would decide on the next treatment. The last things I wanted to deal with on my vacation were unforeseen side effects or complications.

I came home from that appointment dejected and upset (although not as upset as I have been in the past—you get used to bad news after a while). I was lying on the couch when I asked Isabelle to come over and give me a hug. This is the conversation we had:

Me: Isabelle, Mama is getting sicker.

[Silence for a few seconds as she looked at me contemplatively]

Belle: Mommy, how old are you?

Me: I'm forty.

Belle [with no hesitation]: That's old.

Me: No, not really. There are lots of people who live until they're eighty or ninety.

[She looked away from me, staring at the TV for a good long time, and then she turned toward me again and looked me in the eye and said]

Belle: Mommy, you're not gone yet.

I gave Isabelle a big hug then, marveling once again at this child who in other contexts acts like any other four-year-old, but when I need her emotionally, she becomes a sage and speaks as if she has lived before, as if in some part of her bottomless soul she remembers the lessons from a previous life.

33

Insanity

For the first time, I find myself ever closer to a lonely insanity. I endeavor to give voice to the most painful and, some might say, the most humiliating and unflattering aspects of myself as I flounder through the journey that is living with cancer—the rage, jealousy, bitterness, terror, and sorrow. While I write and share the ugliest parts of this journey in a way that I could never verbalize accurately or completely for my own cathartic reasons (among others), I share also because I know that such brute honesty validates the dark emotions of those who feel as I do as they stumble through their own trials, whether they be cancer-related or not. And in that validation, you and I, we, regardless of whether we've ever met in person, find a connection, a oneness in our suffering that speaks to the universal human experience, which transcends class, race, culture, time, and space.

I want you all to know that it is to this connection that I cling as the loneliness of this journey threatens to swallow me. And that is even as I found myself posting pictures on Facebook from our glorious Sicilian vacation—wandering around a snowcapped volcano, the children dancing and twirling through piazza after piazza, exploring two-thousand-year-old ruins under the life-giving Mediterranean sun, basking in the fragrance of blooming blood orange trees, gorging on the freshest of gelatos and granitas. Then the weekend after our return, I flew to Los Angeles sans husband and children to join Cousin N in a little adventure of our own, during which we saw and came within five feet of meeting Oprah. I've loved Oprah since I was a kid, watching her show while I did my homework. I posted pictures of me smiling and having fun and living large.

That's what I'm supposed to do, right? Live as large as I can to show myself and the whole world and the cancer itself (as if it were some sentient being) that it cannot and will never defeat me. *Bullshit!* I call bullshit on myself and everyone else who constructs those façades.

Those pictures only told half-truths, and in that way I was lying; I was being disingenuous. Beneath the sometimes strained smiles and laughter lay the darkness and the ugliness that had come to the forefront of my mind again. Don't misunderstand me—we had a wonderful time in Sicily. It was the first time that I took possession of this family I had created. Until Sicily, I never felt that Mia and Isabelle were truly my children or that we, with Josh, were a family in our own right. My family was the family into which I was born, of course, not these two little people who had their own personalities that I was still trying to understand. And Josh—well, he was my husband, my lover, my best friend, my partner, but not my "family." It was sometime during the many hours we spent in our rented Mercedes station wagon, driving 1300 kilometers around the not-so-small island over eleven days, as we played verbal games, like "I Spy" and "What would you rather have?" (as in "Would you rather have apples or oranges?" "Would you rather live in the city or in the country?"), that I realized that those moments were reminiscent of my own memories with my parents, siblings, and me making long road trips to San Francisco and Las Vegas when I was a child. And weren't these shared memories, together with our joined bloodlines, the heart of what it means to be a family?

And then I wondered about how many more family vacations we would be able to take, how many more crazy adventures we would have, how many more precious memories we would be able to make. And as I answered those questions on the basis of my fears, I could feel the sadness and the bitterness and jealousy mounting and then the pressure to make as many great memories as I could on this vacation,

because this vacation might very well be the only vacation with me
that Mia and Isabelle would ever remember. Therefore, I couldn't be
sad, and I had to push all the cancer stuff out of my mind. But the reality is you can't ever push the cancer stuff out of your mind, not when
you live with metastatic disease, and the harder you try the more present it becomes. Josh felt the same pressures. So we would fight and
then cry. The pictures don't tell that part of the story.

We returned to New York on a Saturday. First thing Monday I had
another abdominal and pelvic MRI and chest CT. I had been off treatment while I was on vacation, so I expected the scans to show growth.
My lung nodules had grown one to two millimeters in the six weeks
since my last scans. But more concerning, my left ovary was enlarged,
which likely meant that cancer had spread to my ovaries. Dr. A.C.
wanted me to see a gynecological oncologist, Dr. B. As soon as I knew
about the enlarged ovary, I started to feel discomfort and pain in the
area—the mind can be so powerful. I couldn't get an appointment
with Dr. B. for another two weeks. Completely unacceptable. I texted
my oncologist, telling him about the growing pain, and asked him to
help. He called her and told her she had to move up the appointment,
and she did.

I did see Oprah and had fun with Cousin N, but mostly I worried
and stressed and cried, playing out every conceivable scenario in my
mind, convinced that disease had spread to my peritoneum, in which
case I had only a few months left, that the cancer while I was off treatment was working its way up my spine and into my brain, that I would
need Gamma Knife radiation, and how would I be able to write everything I want to write for my girls if the cancer was in my brain? And on
and on the thoughts came, and overran my mind, playing on repeat
like some agonizing broken record. Torture that threatened to destroy
me. Insanity.

I could feel the animal panic rising in me; I was being forced by the
gargoyles atop the towering stone walls to walk ever faster toward my
execution, their arrows ever more primed, their stone bodies ready
any second to spring into life. The pain generated by the enlarged
ovary grew worse and worse, to the point where for the first time I was
truly afraid of the pain that will come as I die! What if the doctors can-

not control the pain? What if the narcotics cause hallucinations, making me try to rip off my skin like a patient in a psychiatric ward? I cannot allow my children to see me like that. More torture that threatened to destroy me. More insanity.

I saw my parents and brother while I was in L.A. My father drove me back to their house in Monterey Park, the house where I had lain in ignorant agony as the tumor grew to completely obstruct my colon, where the abdominal pain had been so severe that I asked my father to take me to the local ER at 4:00 in the morning the day of my cousin's wedding. I will forever associate that house with my cancer diagnosis. That was why I hadn't been back in nearly three years. I just couldn't reenter that traumatic place. So I sat in my father's car in the garage long after my parents had gone up, amid myriad dusty, old, long-forgotten boxes that held my high school yearbooks, my speech competition trophies, my childhood and adolescent memories.

I called Josh then and sobbed to him for a long, long time in perhaps the most crazed and hysterical crying fit I've had since I first got sick. Gone was the persona of my philosophical and sagely self who likes to talk about the evolution of the soul and putting one little life in the context of human history. In those moments and in the many moments since, I've been completely absorbed in my own life and my own pain. I told Josh, as I have often told him, that if it weren't for the girls, him, and my promise to him to try to stay alive for as long as possible, I would stop all treatments and let the cancer run its course, living out my days in some other country doing what I have most loved to do all my life, learn a new language. And then when the pain became too much to bear, I would jump off a bridge to put myself out of my misery in much the same way that we euthanize beloved suffering pets; I would do myself that kindness. But I have a husband and children I love, and so I can't do that; I'm not supposed to do that.

In those moments of utter and complete emotional pain, I wanted the irrational and the impossible; I wanted to travel back in time to warn the little girl and the teenager I once was of her fate so she could change it. I wanted the unknowable; I wanted time to be circular rather than linear; I wanted the afterlife to hold the promise of second and third and fourth chances, the opportunity to live this life again and again and again until I could get it just right, until Josh and I could live out all our dreams together. But most of all, I wanted to simply live out this life, also an impossibility, it seems. I never pray for myself, because I think to do so is supremely arrogant and selfish. Why would God—if there is indeed a God and if he does in fact intervene in our lives—spare my life and not the life of an innocent child who deserves to live more than I? I would never dare to suggest to an almighty being that I am somehow more special than others. But in those desperately painful moments, I prayed to a God I'm not sure even exists that I be spared from this cancer. The pictures don't portray this part of the story, either.

I saw Dr. B. in mid-April. After a physical exam, she concluded that my ovary is not cystic and that whatever is growing is doing so from the inside and that it is likely cancer. She said if my metastases were isolated to the ovaries, it would be an easy and obvious choice to do surgery, but since I already had lung metastases, it didn't make sense to remove the ovary, unless of course I found the pain intolerable, in which case she would happily go in and remove that ovary and proba-bly the other one, too. At that point, I didn't think I had enough pain to justify surgery, but even so, after considering her statements for sev-eral minutes, I disagreed.

I went to see Dr. A.C. immediately afterward. I recounted Dr. B.'s conclusions and then said, "I don't agree. I think this surgery could be an opportunity."

"Exactly!" he proclaimed before I had a chance to elaborate.

It gratified me greatly to discover again that Dr. A.C. and I think similarly. He and I both view the probably cancerous tissue in my ovary—we won't know for sure until the ovary is removed and the tissue biopsied—to be valuable. It can be used to update the genetic testing that I'd had done on my primary tumor, the bulk of which still sits frozen at UCLA. I needed to have the surgery as soon as possible so I could be back on treatment that much earlier to slow the growth of the lung nodules. I had also decided to spend my own money and have the live cancer cells implanted in immune-suppressed mice. As-suming the implantation was successful, we would then select the drugs to test on my mice to determine whether those drugs might have any cancer-killing effects when directed at my genetically unique cancer. A courier would be waiting outside the operating room to receive the tissue and drive it to New Jersey, where the lab and mice are. The scientists would implant the mice that night or early the next morning.

There's also the possibility that further chemotherapy will have no impact on my ovaries. It is more likely not to work well in that area, just like on the peritoneum. I don't want the things to get any larger and cause me additional pain, at which point, in order to have surgery, I would have to take at least four weeks off treatment. Surgery seems meant to be now, since I've already been off treatment for four weeks. The window of opportunity is open; I must take advantage of that. Furthermore, I can't help but rationally conclude that it's better to remove whatever cancer one can in order to extend life, particularly when the surgery is low risk and not that invasive.

Although the window of opportunity is open, it is closing fast. I'm convinced that the cancer will spread to my brain next. While we are dealing with my ovaries, the lung mets are growing. Dr. A.C. told me that the probability of the cancer going to my brain is very low. My response: "The probability of the cancer going to my ovaries was low. The probability of it skipping my liver and going to my lungs was relatively low. The probability of me even getting colon cancer at age thirty-seven was low. So I don't fucking care about probabilities. They don't apply to me. So get the surgery scheduled for me ASAP." Yes, this is how I sometimes talk to my oncologist, who takes it all in stride.

It took a couple days of me exchanging late-night texts with Dr. A.C. and bugging him on his cellphone because of Dr. B.'s lack of response, but we finally scheduled the surgery. It will be a laparoscopic bilateral oophorectomy, which in the best-case scenario will take an hour, assuming minimal scar tissue from prior surgeries. Also depending on the amount of scar tissue, Dr. B. will be able to take a look around and see if I have disease on my peritoneum, and then depending on the extent of disease, she will try to remove whatever cancer she sees if she can do so quickly. I will be able to restart treatment a week later.

I made the decision to have surgery within minutes; I had already considered this scenario during the week I waited to see Dr. B. I had already evaluated, processed, and plotted this next step. Plus, I'm by nature a quick decision maker, even when it comes to big, life-changing decisions. I've always trusted my instincts, the seeming signals the universe would send to me. It was no different here. Josh was taken aback by the speed of my decision, unprepared for this sudden new move, as if in some self-protective tactic he had allowed himself to believe and hope that this enlarged ovary was nothing serious.

Another reason I hate hope—it slows down reaction time, it lulls one into complacency; it allows one to live in useless delusion. So, we fought, he arguing that I was being too rash, that any surgery is major, and I arguing that he was constantly living in denial and unprepared to confront reality and that I didn't have the luxury of time to sit around and deliberate; after all, I was simply following through on my promise to him to do everything I could to stay alive for as long as possible because if it were up to me I wouldn't do any of this shit. It was a bad fight, which on top of the stresses of trying to schedule the surgery and the ongoing worry of what will be found during surgery, drove me to the brink. Yet more insanity.

Up to now, I've not written specifically about my and Josh's relationship and how it has weathered the stresses and pressures of cancer. Josh is a much more private person than I am, and I want to respect his need for privacy. All the same, friends do ask me how Josh is doing and how we are doing as a couple. Because in addition to destroying bodies, cancer has an incredible power to destroy relationships, too. The struggle to keep relationships whole and healthy as cancer does its worst is particularly arduous and, for some people, impossible.

A friend who died within two years of her diagnosis told me she sometimes felt like her husband and she were two ghosts living in the same house, pale shadows of their former happy selves, circling each other, not knowing what to say, disconnected from each other and the rest of the world, so lonely and isolated in their individual suffering. I now know what she meant. Because Josh and I are on sharply divergent paths—mine leads toward death and whatever awaits, and his toward a new life without me but with the children and a new wife. My greatest fears are a painful death and not doing everything I want to do before I die. His greatest fear is going on without me. I am angry at him for the happy life I know he will rebuild after I am gone. He is angry at me for getting sick and dying. I feel endless guilt for having married him and dooming him to be a widower at such a young age, and the children to be motherless. He feels endless guilt for not being able to save me. And in all of our fear, anger, guilt, and sadness we feel alone, and so impotent in our inability to help each other.

That's how we are doing, even as we love and need each other more than ever before.

I cope by planning. I make lists of all our expenses and how and when they're paid so when I'm not here Josh will know what to do. I talk to his boss secretly to tell him what I want for Josh's career. I ask my beloved contractor to do me the favor of helping Josh with things around the apartment. I talk to the administrators and teachers at the girls' school so they can help the girls get into good high schools so that some of the pressure is taken off of Josh. I'm building a beautiful home for him and the girls. I'm getting them a dog. Josh would tell me he doesn't care about any of those things, that he just wants me. Sadly, that's really the only thing I can't give him.

In the midst of all this craziness, I went to get a routine dental cleaning from my periodontist. I had X-rays done because one tooth was feeling a little strange. The X-rays showed that I have five cavities. Five freaking cavities! I've never had so many cavities. It really started to feel like everything was going wrong, one more damn thing to deal with, something else in my body falling apart. Discovering these cavities just about pushed me over the edge. I called my longtime dentist, Dr. D., and asked for an emergency appointment. In light of my upcoming surgery, I had to get these cavities dealt with ASAP. I hadn't seen Dr. D. in almost two years because I had been lazy about making the trek to his new office, but he is the best dentist ever, very anal and very enthusiastic about teeth. He wasn't going to see patients the next day, but for me he would make an exception. So I went in.

He told me based on my X-rays, he thought two of the teeth might need root canals. *Root canals.* He also said that the pattern of decay was consistent with someone who has chronic dry mouth brought on by chemo and other types of medications. The decay in those two teeth proved to be very deep, but it had not touched the roots, so no root canals. What a relief. Dr. D. said, "You are very lucky." I would have laughed if I didn't have a bunch of dental instruments in my mouth. The notion of me being lucky was ludicrous. And then as I lay there with Dr. D. diligently sculpting my new filling like he was Michelangelo, I realized that I was really lucky in a sense to have him and so many other people in my life who are there to take care of me and my family, from my oncologist to my internist to my construction team to my many friends and family. What did I ever do to deserve such good and kind people from all walks of my life?

Josh isn't so into talking and sharing as I am, and so I don't think he gives people a chance to offer him support. Typical guy. And sadly, I don't think caregivers get as much attention or support as cancer patients, even though their suffering and loneliness are just as great.

34

Chipper

On May 20, I had my laparoscopic oophorectomy (which is a fun word to say). My left ovary was about two to three centimeters bigger than it should have been. An intraoperative biopsy was performed on it and confirmed that the growth (which was inside the ovary) was metastatic colon cancer. About one cubic centimeter of that cancerous tissue was immediately handed over to a courier for transport to a laboratory across the river in New Jersey where portions of it were successfully implanted into five mice, a very good number, I am told.

My mice have since been moved down to Baltimore, to the main laboratory. I will know in a couple weeks whether the graft of my cancer cells into these mice has taken hold and, if so, they will be cloned for personalized experimentation. While the right ovary looked normal, out of an abundance of caution, it was also removed, together with my fallopian tubes. I'm losing parts at a pretty good clip now. As the final pathology would later reveal, appearances were deceptive and the right ovary tested positive for metastatic colon cancer as well. All else looked normal in the abdomen, including all organs located therein as well as my peritoneum. Forty milliliters of ascites—fluid—were found, however. The word "ascites" terrifies me; I often hear it associated with end-stage cancer, where hundreds of milliliters can build up in the abdomen as the cancer overruns the body. Fortunately, the pathology report declared the ascites to be negative. The surgeon also flooded my abdominal cavity with saline, then withdrew it and had it tested for cancer, something that was also done during my post-HIPEC diagnostic laparoscopy. That saline was negative for cancer, as it was in October 2014. If indeed there is no cancer in my abdominal cavity, then it certainly indicates that the HIPEC surgical treatment from March 2014 has withstood the cancer assault well.

It was the best news I could have asked for under the circumstances, minus the cancerous right ovary. But then again, metastases to the ovaries are often bilateral, and besides, what is the difference really between having one cancerous ovary and two? That's how you start to think when you've been living with metastatic cancer for a while: Oh, what's the big deal with another tumor? Oh, what's another affected organ?

My surgical recovery was about as uneventful and painless as they come. I don't think I even took one Percocet. Surgery started around 1:00. I was home by eight that evening, and all I showed for those hours were a hunched-over stance when I stood and three tiny bandages covering three tiny holes. Oh, and I had trouble peeing for the first twelve hours, an aftereffect of the catheter used during surgery. I marvel at how they were able to remove two organs, one of which was grossly enlarged, through those tiny holes. In case you are wondering how exactly that was possible, the surgeon chopped them up. And to prevent cancer from spreading everywhere (which is what would have happened if she had cut them where they lay), she detached the ovaries, lifted them into a bag she had inserted under my skin, performed all the chopping inside that bag, and then sucked the entire bag out through one of the three tiny holes. Medical science is simply amazing.

I continue to be baffled by how either the scans missed this massive growth in my left ovary all this time or the cancer managed to grow to the point of detection in the span of six weeks, which was the period between my last sets of abdominal MRIs. The doctors can't answer that question, either. Really reassuring . . . My oncologist is less inclined to believe that the cancer grew that rapidly and so is thinking that the scans missed it. And obviously, the cancer in the ovaries was resistant to months and months of treatment. Also very reassuring . . . This time I am really being facetious.

I restarted treatment ten days after the surgery. The three treatments I've had since the surgery have been uneventful. I have been experiencing pain in my hips and knees. I cannot determine if the pain is bone- or muscle-related. Perhaps it's attributable to the sudden loss of all the estrogen that was once produced by my ovaries. Perhaps it is due to weight gain from the steroids and my failure to go to the gym for months and months. Or perhaps I can blame it on all the hours I spend on my feet now taking the dog out in my efforts to house-train him.

The five weeks after the surgery found me pretty much MIA from social media, and to a lesser degree, my friends and family. Unlike prior periods of reclusiveness, this one was not because I was in some dark cancer-induced malaise. For the last nearly three years, I have always chosen to confront my disease head-on, to live it, embrace it, forcing myself to walk through the fires and feel the pain, in the belief that I would emerge from the other side stronger and wiser. But not this time. Running and hiding was what I wanted. It was what I needed as part of some kind of mental and emotional recuperation.

My little bichon frise puppy, Chipper (named after the Atlanta Braves player Chipper Jones—Chipper came from Atlanta and Josh is a fan of the Braves), facilitated that objective. Two days after my first postsurgical treatment, as I was crashing from the steroidal high, Josh, the girls, and I drove to the airport, searching for an obscure building in the bowels of La Guardia, to which little Chipper was brought. He was adorable, all white fluff with dark black eyes and velvety, floppy ears. And I was terrified as I clutched his crate in the passenger seat, wondering how I was going to have the energy to take care of yet another living thing, and a living thing that was even more foreign to me than a newborn baby had once been, no less. He came home and almost immediately pooped on our wood floor as I lunged to place a wee-wee pad under his butt; I wasn't fast enough. That night he cried incessantly, waking me up every hour. I would take him out of his crate, he would suddenly run from me (a sure sign that he was about to do his business), I would run after him with a wee-wee pad, he would pee or poop not on the wee-wee pad. I would clean up the mess and put him back in his crate, and then the cycle would repeat an hour or two later, and on and on this seemed to go over the next few days. I was exhausted thanks to the sleep deprivation and the treatment, on the verge of hysterical tears, convinced that I had made a serious error in judgment by getting this dog and wondering if the breeder would take him back if I begged.

House training was made much more difficult by the fact that we live in an apartment building and by the vet's directive that I not take Chipper outside (or that at least I prevent his paws from touching the ground) because he wasn't fully vaccinated yet, and it would be another seven weeks before he would be. The streets are apparently rife with deadly canine diseases. As per my dog trainer's recommendation, I kept the dog in his crate and would carry him out on a leash every couple hours into the stairwell, where I laid down a couple wee-wee pads. With the leash, I kept him on the pads, but Chipper refused to do as I wanted. He would sit, lie down, and roll around. I would sit on a step while he lay on a pad, bored, waiting. I spent hours in that stairwell, fruitlessly waiting. And apparently, Chipper was waiting, too, because invariably the moment I put him back in his crate, he would pee or poop. And so it went.

After a week of this, I decided to willfully disregard the vet's instructions, and I carried Chipper outside—I didn't know this, but when you carry a dog, he won't eliminate on you, just as he would never eliminate on his mother. And miracle of miracles, he peed and pooped almost immediately! I decided that venturing outside with him within a limited area where there are few dogs and most of the dogs are from my building and are therefore more trustworthy healthwise involved minimal risk, and a risk that I had to assume because my sanity hung in the balance.

Once I started walking Chipper outside, I discovered something extraordinary, at least it was extraordinary for someone like me, who comes from an animal-hating family. I learned that people, at least most people, *love* dogs. When my children were babies, I got the occasional smile from a stranger gazing at my adorable offspring; on the whole, though, few people care about cute babies. But a puppy? Unbelievable! Young, old, black, white, brown, businessmen, garbage collectors, construction workers, Goth girls, tough guys—everyone from all ages and all walks of life and every part of the world has stopped to pet and play with my dog. We engage in conversations about their dogs at home, about how they are still grieving their dearly departed dogs, about how they wish they could have a dog.

My nurse-practitioner (another one of those fanatics who prefers dogs over babies), upon learning I had gotten a puppy, insisted that I bring him to the cancer center when I came for treatment. I was nervous about potential complaints, as was my oncologist. But my nurse-practitioner blew off Dr. A.C.'s concerns and told me to do it anyhow. I was concerned about leaving Chipper home alone for so long, so I did as I was told, carrying him in a little bag that I tried to hide as I sneaked past the security guard. The waiting room was packed with at least fifty people, as usual. But what was not usual was the sudden burst of energy and life that swept through the room when people realized there was a puppy in their midst. Staff came out of the internal offices and exam rooms, squealing with delight. Patients and their caregivers smiled and stared, and some even rushed over to pet and hold the dog. And little Chipper took it all in stride, basking in the attention and then sleeping on me as I received my infusion. He did not once bark or cry or do anything remotely troubling while at the cancer center. I should mention though that there were a few people in the waiting room who did not look at all excited to see the dog. In fact, I might even characterize their expressions as ones of incredulity and disgust. They were the Chinese people, those of my parents' generation. I could relate.

House training is going well, now that I know what to do. Chipper stopped crying during the night after three days and now sleeps through without incident. People told me having a puppy was like having a newborn baby. I don't agree at all. When I don't want to deal with Chipper, I stick him in his crate. He sleeps through the night and doesn't require endless breast feeding. I don't need to change any diapers. He doesn't cry or bark. When I take him out, I don't have to bring tons of baby paraphernalia with me. He is much, much easier than a baby.

And the best part about him is his simplicity, the complete lack of complication. I have no expectations of him to be a Rhodes Scholar or concert violinist one day, and he doesn't chafe under or resent my demands. We don't have a difficult relationship in which I have to lecture him about the value of money and how I can't buy him a toy whenever he wants. He has truly basic needs that are generally very easy to satisfy and that, I've discovered, I am capable of fulfilling. And he loves unconditionally, with a purity that is in its own way quite beautiful and inspiring. It is in the performance of our daily, mesmerizing rituals—me squatting with a plastic bag in hand to pick up his waste, me tossing a squeaky frog as he eagerly waits to give chase, me brushing out the tangles in his snowy coat—that I find that he and his simplicity shield me from what I don't want to deal with right now, and he allows me to continue with my pretense for as long as I want. And within those rituals, there is no cancer, no life, no death, no future, no past, not even that day or hour or even minute, not even Josh or the girls or me; there is just that second, and then the next and then the next. And there is just him.

35

Courage and Love

ho has more courage? (1) The cancer patient who presses on with grueling treatments that are of dubious benefit in the infinitesimal hope that they will prolong life until something better comes along? or (2) The cancer patient who simply walks away, choosing to feel good for as long as she can and then seeking palliative treatments only to mitigate pain before the inevitable happens?

This is a question that has plagued me for nearly as long as I've known that I have cancer. As you may have surmised, I put a great deal of weight on courage and bravery. I want to be remembered as a courageous person, one who, instead of running from cancer and death and begging for my life like a wild, crazed animal, stood there and stared them down, all the while acknowledging and embracing the reality and my fear, anger, and sadness, a stance reflective of an aspirational inner strength, dignity, grace, and beauty. But which path produces that result? Based on how we as a society seem to love sports stories and movies about protagonists overcoming impossible odds, I believe the general consensus and more popular view is number 1. I understand that—the long-suffering patient who endures so much to spend just one more day with her loved ones, even if it comes at an incredible emotional and physical toll. But then again, it takes tremendous courage to stop all treatments and to let the disease run its course, because then gone is any semblance of a safety net as that person invites death to quicken its arrival. Isn't that person then truly staring death in the face? Isn't that person then choosing death on her own terms with dignity and grace? Or is that person truly a coward, a horrible wife and mother, too weakened, defeated, and exhausted to fight any longer, not even for the faintest promise of one more day with her beloved children, handicapped by an inferior love that does have limits?

Or maybe the answer to that question is personal to each individual, based on a subjective determination of which path is easier—if there is such a thing—and that true courage goes to the person who takes the path more difficult for that person.

For me, the easier path, the path of less resistance, is number 2. And I suppose that if I take that path, then I am a coward for not choosing to stay on and "fight" like the "warrior" I'm supposed to be and once was. I hate the rhetoric of war that pervades the cancer world, even though I once used it liberally. With fighting and war, there is a winner and a loser. Will you judge me then a loser when I die because I succumbed to my disease? Will you judge me a loser if I simply choose to stop treatment and to stop actively "fighting"? If you do, so be it.

It seems that I have come to the end of the road of tolerable treatment options, and therefore there is a particular urgency in my coming to an answer to this question. I had scans in mid-June and received my results a few days later. While my lungs are overall stable (one tumor's notable shrinkage and another tumor's growth, with all other lung tumors remaining stable), the abdominal and pelvic MRI showed an enlarged peritoneal lymph node as well as a questionable spot around my uterus. The latter may be postsurgical "stuff," but it is impossible for us to know without another surgery. In addition, my CEA continues to rise. Dr. A.C. is not a fan of the current treatment (irinotecan and Avastin). Who could blame him? This recycling of prior drugs was really a last-ditch effort by me to try the only remaining likely effective treatment available in the hope that these drugs' prior use had not as yet desensitized my cancer cells to them. Dr. A.C. believes that continuing with the irinotecan and Avastin may make us feel good because it seems like we are doing "something," but he doesn't think that we would actually be doing anything beneficial, at least not for much longer. There remain two FDA-approved drugs for treating colorectal cancer, one of which is so toxic I swore I would never take it and the other of which is highly unimpressive and tantamount to a waste of time.

Dr. A.C. then asked me if I wanted to do something "crazy." I had to hear what his "crazy" idea was, of course. Because he doesn't believe that single-agent immunotherapy will work with the specifics of my tumor biology, he thinks we need to attempt combined immunotherapy, and the drugs he has in mind and has access to are ipilimumab (brand name Yervoy) and nivolumab (brand name Opdivo). Both are FDA-approved drugs that have been used with success to treat metastatic melanoma. Each drug forces two different receptors on cells that constitute part of our immune system to identify cancer cells as unwanted and thereby allow the immune system to kill them. Dr. A.C. would also throw in a little radiation therapy (probably directed at that peritoneal lymph node) to trigger an initial immune response and jump-start the immune system. This would be done "off trial," meaning outside of a clinical trial.

Sounds exciting, huh? Crazy always sounds exciting, but then there are certain complications. First, there's the matter of getting the drugs for off-label use, since the FDA hasn't approved them for colorectal cancer. Dr. A.C. seems to have some connections with the pharmaceutical companies, though, so I think he would succeed, although he himself said it wouldn't be easy. More concerning to me is that the use of the drugs—known as anti-PD1 and anti-CTLA4 inhibitors, respectively—would preclude me from future clinical trials that include the use of these or any other anti-PD1 and anti-CTLA4 inhibitors. Of course, this is only a concern if I want to participate in clinical trials.

Dr. A.C. said he would probably opt for a clinical trial over "crazy." He wants whatever trial I do to be one with combination immunotherapy. He says he will talk to his contacts at Memorial Sloan Kettering, Columbia-Presbyterian, and Johns Hopkins, all places that have strong immunotherapy departments. If I want to go for trials, I will also have to do the research myself. It's a daunting task.

Most of the trials available are Phase I trials, trials where the experimental drug is being tested for safety, not effectiveness. That's a frightening thought, isn't it? I've heard people say that the odds of a clinical trial working are 5 percent. I think they're much less than that, more like 0.1 percent.

Josh believes it's worth "fighting" based on that 0.1 percent. I don't agree. Why should I allow myself to be treated like a lab rat, poked and prodded, monitored, scrutinized, suffering who-the-hell-knows what side effects? Why should I diminish the quality of whatever time I have left with my children when the chance of success is so small? Why bother when the endgame is the same?

I'm tired. I'm so very, very tired, so tired that I don't want to do anything at all, not "crazy" stuff or clinical trials. For those of you who don't live with metastatic cancer, who haven't undergone all the surgeries and treatments, can you possibly understand the depth of my fatigue—physical, emotional, and spiritual? I don't think so. It's the kind of exhaustion that tests not just any courage I have but also the tremendous love I have for my husband and children.

I'm tired of feeling the strain of living as normal a life as possible under the constant threat of death. Of combating the jealousy and anger upon seeing the grandmother who has the privilege of taking her grandson to school and the envy upon hearing another mother's carefree laughter with her friends. Of feeling the hatred of the woman whom Josh will marry after I am gone, who will live in the home that I designed and have the honor of raising my beautiful children, who will hang her dresses in my closet, who will steal the life that should have been mine. Of feeling the sadness at the thought of Mia sitting in her weekly violin lesson without me there for her to glance at once in a while for reassurance and encouragement. Of worrying and planning and more worrying and more planning. This is the text of an email that I wrote to Mia's violin teacher, a manifestation of my sadness, worry, and planning:

Hi A,

I think I told you at some point that I have metastatic cancer, incurable and likely terminal. When you told us this week about your violin teacher and how she got you through the first 7 years of your violin life before she died of cancer, it was obvious how much she meant to you and no doubt how much you meant to her. Anyhow, it got me thinking, so just bear with me as you read this.

While everyone tells me I need to be positive, I'm a realist and a planner. You are so young so probably some of what I say won't resonate with you yet, but I will do my best to explain. What makes me the saddest about dying is the thought of Mia learning during her lessons and me not sitting right next to her, watching her. The thought of her performing on a bigger stage and me not being there in the front row to cheer her on breaks my heart into a million little pieces. The image of her practicing by herself without me there to push and yell and demand and hug and teach (not the violin but about life) both worries and saddens me. Who will and can replace me? Who can nurture her musically and otherwise as I can? The answer is no one. No one can possibly love my children as much as I do, not even their father. So the best thing I can do is to line up as many people as I can to be there for them in the different aspects of their lives. That's what I want to talk to you about.

While Mia's father is very musically talented, he works a lot and I don't see him fulfilling the music role left empty by my death. What I'm asking of you is for you—as much as you are able—to take Mia under your wing, to look out for her musically, to guide her and push her when she needs it, to advise her in getting into music programs and, if/when the time comes, find a new teacher for her.

I know Mia has musical talent, how much I really don't know. It doesn't really matter to me how much talent she has. What matters is that she develops the talent she has. I don't want it to go to waste. Plus, I think she really enjoys playing and likes to perform. She's one of those people that keeps her feelings to herself, which I don't think is a healthy coping mechanism. It is my hope that music becomes an emotional outlet for her, a way for her to deal with the grief from my loss and the other hardships that will inevitably come into her life.

How much you want to and can help Mia is of course up to you. I will understand if you can't do much at all beyond the weekly lessons. But if you want to be more involved in her life and get to know us better, the invitation is always out there. We live right around the cor-

ner from the school. Mia likes you, and obviously you are good at re-
lating to little girls.

So thanks for having taught Mia as much as you have (and me,
too). You've no idea, but the lessons are a highlight of my week. I always wanted a musical education, but my parents were too poor to
give me one. And thanks for reading all this and putting up with my
emotional outburst.

It is because of my jealousy and hate and worry and love that I have
threatened Josh with murder from the grave if he were to ever favor
future children over our children, even monetarily. I made him promise that he would not move out of this apartment that I have spent so
much time and energy renovating for my children because the Slutty
Second Wife demands that, to banish all traces of me. A friend told me
about a little boy who lost his mother to cancer at age one; subsequently, his father remarried, and now, four years later, that boy calls
this woman Mom. That story made me cringe and incited hysteria.

As I write all this, I know how unhinged I sound. I'm crazy. Josh
would tell you I was crazy to begin with and cancer has made me cra-
zier.

Poor Josh has to put up with my hysterics, my anger, my sadness,
my tears, my darkness. Josh is tired, too. He's tired of living under this
black cloud. And out of love for him, I want to die sooner rather than
later. I want to set him and the children free. I want him to have a normal, happy life again. And no doubt, his family wants the same for
him. I am a burden. I don't want to be an embarrassment to him at
family gatherings, me with my ravaged skin and body—oh, poor Josh,
they must all think. It will be a lot better for him when my presence is
gone and he has someone else with whom to share the rest of his life,
someone who will help him heal and forget the pain.

So now you understand what I am wrestling with. Is it more courageous to continue or to stop? Is it more loving to leave or to stay? I still
don't know.

36

Hate

I used to not hate people. But now I hate people. Can you guess who I hate the most?

It isn't the grandmother who has the privilege of taking her grandson to violin lesson, the one I always see when I come out of Mia's lesson. No doubt that is a privilege she doesn't even fully appreciate.

It isn't even the old lady with a cane who criticized me for taking a seat at the front of the bus reserved for the disabled and thereby forcing a man hobbling down the aisle to take another seat a few feet away—I shut her up when I screamed at her that I have Stage IV cancer and yanked at the neck of my T-shirt to show her and everyone else on the bus the unmistakable bump on my chest under which lies my mediport. I wanted to scream something about my legal blindness, too, making me disabled on yet another level and entirely entitled to that seat in ways she could not possibly understand, and that she should go fuck herself. But the presence of my older daughter beside me stopped me. (My poor children. They have been so traumatized by me and no doubt will carry with them confusing and humiliating memories of their angry mother acting like a stark-raving lunatic on this and many other occasions. I hope they will understand that the rage was rooted in a deep love for them.)

Then there was the tall, well-dressed woman who made some snide comment at me when Chipper got away on his leash and therefore interfered with her self-absorbed rush along the broad sidewalk outside my building. I wanted to chase her down and punch her again and again and again, until all the rage inside me found an escape. I wanted to claw her eyes out. I wanted to strangle her to death. I still do. Criminal charges, imprisonment, life sentences, none of them matter in those moments of fury. But my children were with me, so I just let the incident pass. Even though I wanted to kill that woman, I don't hate her the most, either.

Nor is it all the other mothers I know and don't know who get to attend back-to-school nights and listen to the new teachers talk about homework routines, all without worrying about who exactly is going to make sure their children do homework after they die and more broadly, about how the hell their children are not going to become totally fucked up in light of their mother's death.

It isn't even mothers who have been cured of Stage I or II or III cancer.

Don't get me wrong—I hate all of these people to some degree, at least in the abstract. But the people I hate above all others are the mothers who were diagnosed with Stage IV cancer and who somehow were cured, who for some unknown reason escaped the death sentence. I find myself asking a God that never answers my questions—Why? Why them and not me? But that question seems inconsequential when I think of my children. I would sacrifice myself for my children a million times over. Are those women's children somehow more deserving of a mother than mine are? My children are incredible little people. Mia is so smart and inquisitive and musically gifted. Isabelle is so compassionate and funny and graceful. If those mothers ever deigned to believe that their lives are more valuable than mine or that their children are more deserving of a mother than mine, I would indeed kill them in cold blood.

What I have written here is perhaps the darkest thing I have ever written, for I am writing about rage, hatred, and violence. I truly believe that such feelings are universal parts of our human experience, brought on by such mundane things as being a mother or living in a place like New York City, the negative by-products of our social interactions and innate tendencies, which are heightened and exacerbated by high-stress conditions like cancer. But such negativity is often unacknowledged because no one wants to talk about something so ugly and unflattering; no one wants to be uncomfortable, embarrassed, ashamed.

But I seem to have lost whatever social graces would have told me to be uncomfortable, embarrassed, or ashamed. I don't care anymore, because I am dying. My oncologist pretty much told me so after the last scans in mid-September. The radiation-immunotherapy combination was a colossal failure. Growth everywhere—in the lungs, in the abdomen, in the pelvis. The worst scans I've ever had. He kept describing new and bigger tumors. It was so awful I couldn't even bring myself to read the scan reports, I, who like to think I'm so smart and should read everything. Dr. A.C. said I have a year without treatment. Given that I've exhausted the first, second, and third lines of treatment, whatever options remain are not going to extend my life much beyond that. And there's always the possibility that treatment, mostly experimental at this point, could make me so sick that it would in fact shorten my life.

Please spare me the platitudes like "Only God knows your expiration date" and "Doctors don't know." Doctors certainly can make a better-educated guess than I can based on their professional experience. And I also don't want to hear the trite "We are all dying."

For a week after the scans I moved through the world in a daze. How could I still be shocked by anything after three years of this shit? I wondered. The daze was worsened by sleep deprivation and intense abdominal and pelvic pain that was most certainly the ever-growing tumors making themselves felt. And yet, I still moved, even though my movements were clumsy.

How did I still manage to walk the dog and get the kids ready for school and sit there and oversee Mia's violin practice? How did I go to a barbecue at Josh's boss's house and smile and act normal? How did I take my children to birthday parties and make Costco runs? How did I

move us back into our home as we finished our months-long apartment combination project? How could I do any of this even as I felt the
life inside of me getting smaller, as I slipped ever closer to death?

Instinct, I suppose. Muscle memory. A powerful sense of obligation. An immensely practical nature, most of all. After I left Dr. A.C.'s
office, I called my sister to tell her the news. Without tears, I told her
that as much as she had not wanted to talk about this, we had to start
talking about "it" now, that she needed to prepare to become my children's surrogate mother, that I would rather she be their surrogate
mother over any random woman Josh married. She would need to be
the one to make sure the kids did their homework and practiced their
instruments; she would need to collect and present to Josh extracur-
ricular activity and summer camp options; she would need to super-
vise the running of the household. Unspoken was the understanding
that she would provide that female emotional support my children
will desperately need. I told her that I had already determined a short
list of friends (and mothers) who would support and help her (since
she doesn't have children of her own), women who would advise her
as necessary. I told her that perhaps this was all meant to be, that her
only sister dying will now afford her the opportunity to experience a
unique brand of motherhood. As much as she hadn't wanted to discuss any of this because she didn't want me to die, she agreed.

We talked about how she could move closer (Queens seems too
far), how she and my brother would divide the responsibility of caring
for our aging parents, how she might possibly move into my apartment temporarily to ease the transition. If there is one thing about the
family into which I was born that I am very proud of, it is that we are
incredibly practical people. No matter how horrible and tragic something is, we always take care of what needs to be taken care of. There
is no emotional withering, no debilitating depression. Our impoverished immigrant roots taught us survival skills that are fundamental to
our very beings. This is an attitude, an approach, a worldview that I
hope the girls, despite their comparatively privileged upbringing, will
have somehow inherited from me.

Josh was devastated. *Stop it,* I thought. How is it possible to still feel
devastated after three years of this, after receiving bad news time and

time again? We comforted each other in the wee hours of the morning, after waking from our brief, exhausted slumber. I forced him to tell me his fears. How would he manage to be a single parent while also maintaining the career that means so much to him? Who could possibly run the household like I do? When should he stop working to be with me? I did my best to address all his fears. I've spent three years planning for my death. I have many contingency plans. Many lists in my head. Many things to write down. Many instructions to issue. If I could, I would handpick Josh's second wife, too, but unfortunately, I haven't gotten around to establishing that contingency plan yet.

I told Josh that I want to be cremated, my ashes to be spread in the Pacific Ocean. I decided on the Pacific Ocean while I stayed at my brother's house this past summer, as I sat in his backyard staring down into the ocean that lies between the landmass where I was born and the one where I lived my improbable life. I told him I want my memorial service to be held at the church we've been going to since Mia demanded we start going over a year ago. I told him I want it to be held three months after I die; three months is enough time for people to make travel arrangements and soon enough to allow Josh and my family to grieve, and then I want them to move on afterward. I want him to ask Mia's violin teacher to perform at the service. I told him who to ask to help with the planning of the service and showed him where old pictures of me can be found. He spent a weekend crying over those faded photographs, bemoaning the unfairness of it all.

I spent the weekend rearranging our chaotic stuff into our new, expanded closets, replacing our old dinnerware with the dishes I just bought, reorganizing spices, cleaning, planning, thinking, and planning some more.

When Dr. A.C. gave me that dim prognosis, I knew I wanted more than a year. I needed more time to plan, to live, to mother. My children need me for as many days as I can give them. Weeks of no chemotherapy had left me feeling pretty good, so I knew I could withstand more treatment.

And so I asked a friend to help me schedule an appointment for that coming week with a prominent GI oncologist in Washington, D.C. (Dr. M.), someone who had helped me with a fundraiser a couple years ago, but whom I had never seen as a patient. If I had gone through regular channels, I would have had to wait six weeks. I got an appointment for the coming Thursday.

I called Memorial Sloan Kettering for an appointment with an oncologist (Dr. V.) I had seen a couple times before for second opinions. She is young and therefore not one of the big names at MSK, but I have always liked her and wanted above all else access to MSK's clinical trials. I had already decided that whatever clinical trials I would do, I would not travel, not unless there was an amazingly promising trial. I wasn't going to waste whatever valuable time I had left with my family traveling constantly for something that was highly unlikely to work. MSK is the leading cancer center in the country, and fortunately for me, it is only a thirty-five-minute subway ride away. Dr. V. had a last-minute cancellation just hours before I was to board a train for D.C. I took it.

Instinctively, I felt the need to obtain other opinions. Dr. A.C. was offering me Lonsurf and Stivarga, the last two drugs approved for colorectal cancer. Dr. V. identified those drugs, but she also offered me a spot in a clinical trial. It is a Phase II trial (meaning that the experimental drug has been tested for safety) involving a chemotherapy agent called SGI-110 that is administered in combination with irinotecan, a chemotherapy drug I've had lots of. Patients are randomized into two arms, one involving SGI-110 and irinotecan, and the other involving either Lonsurf or Stivarga (patient's choice). Even if the patient is randomized into the latter arm, once Lonsurf or Stivarga fails, he or she is assigned to the other arm, so the patient receives the experimental drug sooner or later.

The next morning I saw Dr. M. Despite the unfamiliar environment, it was a relief to see him. He is such a kind man with a wonderful bedside manner, but he also knows what he's talking about. He reassured me. First, he asked me how I was doing emotionally; he knew how I was inside by looking at the scans, but he wanted to know how I was doing in a deeper way. I told him that I was exhausted, that I was tired of making decisions, that I wanted someone I trusted to just tell me what to do.

Dr. M. understood my exhaustion. He took out a piece of paper

and started writing down exactly what I should do: Caris genetic testing of my ovarian tumor from the surgery in May. Updated testing has
a 10 percent chance of helping me determine future clinical trials. He
would take care of it for me if I handled the paperwork, since he can
ask for testing beyond the standard course. Lonsurf and Stivarga have
a 40 percent effectiveness rate for an average of six months, with some
patients experiencing quite a long tail. They both offer stability, not
shrinkage. Stivarga, despite what the blogosphere and the Internet say,
is not so horrible, especially when dosed appropriately—he starts at
120 milligrams. He administers Lonsurf with Avastin. No Avastin with
Stivarga. Choosing between the two is just a question of what side effects I'm willing to tolerate more—nausea and fatigue versus hand-
and-foot syndrome. He knows of the SGI-110 trial and thinks it's
"reasonable" for me to do, and I should allow the randomization gods
to take one decision away from me.

As for how much time I have, he doesn't know. I'm not in any immediate danger. He asked me if I've ever seen my scans. I told him I've
always been afraid to look. He walked me through my scans to illus-
trate the point that I don't have that much disease. We discussed where
my disease was more dangerous, in the lungs or the peritoneum. In
other words, Where will the disease actually kill me? I have always
been afraid of peritoneal disease because my impression is that it
grows so quickly. He said that if he had to choose, he would say peritoneal is more dangerous, not because of the rate of progression but
because of the implications for quality of life. Peritoneal disease causes
bowel blockages, which have a tremendous impact on quality of life
(i.e., pain and the inability to eat and drink). However, at that point,
artificial food administered through IV becomes an option. The disease in my lungs is still small, a centimeter here, a centimeter there.
But once that disease grows large enough, my lungs will fail and I will
die. There is no artificial means to get around failing lungs.

My meeting with Dr. M. was the best oncological appointment I
have ever had. Speaking to him made me realize how I had been having misgivings about Dr. A.C. for a while, how he could never answer
my questions or seemed to always defer my questions. Dr. A.C. was
the kind of doctor with whom I could have a collaborative relation-

ship, the kind of doctor I could text and email any time of day. But I don't want or need that anymore. Dr. M. condemned him for allowing me to go on the radiation and immunotherapy combination. He was furious because I have now burned a bridge to go on trials for other immunotherapy drugs involving similar agents. I was well aware of this risk, as was Dr. A.C., but he seemed to brush it off and so did I. I now have so much regret for going along with Dr. A.C.'s "crazy" idea. As a friend told me, though, it's impossible to go through this cancer journey without having regrets, given the number of decisions we have to make at every turn. But I don't think the detour will make much of a difference ultimately. I'm still going to die.

I went in to see Dr. V. to sign the consent to enter the SGI-110 trial and to tell her that I would be switching my care to her and MSK, even after the trial. I have always been put off by the institutional nature of MSK, the long waits, the lines to enter the elevator, the seeming impersonal nature of it all, but I don't care anymore. I want the institutional support. I believe that I'm looking at months rather than years now, and so I want an institution like MSK to be behind me.

I'm feeling much better now that there is a plan, and recent events have brought me a strange kind of peace, and calm. My abdominal pain is gone. I went lap swimming for the first time in years, and even though I've always struggled to breathe with the proper technique, I learned that day with the help of a friend and a stranger swimming in the neighboring lane.

Despite what I just wrote, I don't hate any of you.

2017

37

Faith, a Lesson of History

It meant that I was closer to the end, but I didn't care—I was glad to see 2016 go. With it I felt a great deal of bitchiness go, too. I would rededicate myself to making memories for Mia and Belle.

The Chilean writer Isabel Allende (most famous for her novel *The House of the Spirits*), in her memoir *Paula,* tells the story of her extraordinary life to her daughter Paula, as she lies in a porphyria-induced coma from which she will never awaken. I read *Paula* more than fifteen years ago, and yet a series of sentiments recorded on page 23 have never left me, and they come back to me now more powerfully than ever. Allende tells her daughter of her past—a thing she calls her "innermost garden, a place not even my most intimate lover has glimpsed." "Take it, Paula," she tells her, "perhaps it will be of some use to you, because I fear that yours no longer exists, lost somewhere during your long sleep—and no one can live without memories."

I am a lover of memories, of the past, of history. I majored in history in college, studying American, Chinese, European, African, social, economic, political, and cultural history. I find fascinating how some unique, charismatic figures, like Jesus Christ and Chairman Mao, and revolutionary innovators, like Thomas Edison and Steve Jobs, altered the course of human history. The rest of us are merely swept along by the tide of events set in motion by others, past and present, and by events that are brought about by forces that are entirely beyond our control (i.e., God, Mother Nature, or the randomness of the universe, which brings about things like natural disasters and illness, depending on one's religious and philosophical views).

It is the stories of the rest of us that I find most intriguing and valuable—the story of the black Caribbean woman who fled her abusive husband for a New York City shelter with her three children, the tale of how an American World War II POW survived months alone drifting at sea and then years of torture by the Japanese, the saga of the incredible will to live of members of a Uruguayan rugby team whose plane crashed into the Andes in 1972, the unlikely story of one woman's ability to live fifteen years after being diagnosed with metastatic colon cancer. There are so many stories. Indeed, the truth that has been lived by our fellow human beings is much more inspiring than any yarn woven by the greatest storytellers.

But Allende reminds me that there is value in our individual memories, our own past, our own history; after all, what are we but the products of all our experiences? Rather than looking without to find inspiration, strength, and hope, sometimes we must look within ourselves to discover and discern our own stories. There are, after all, miracles in there. Of course, looking within is much more difficult, for we must confront our painful mistakes, our fears, our weaknesses, our insecurities, our ugliness.

When I was first diagnosed with cancer, Josh read my surgical and pathology reports what seemed like a hundred times. I could barely manage to get through my surgical report once without being nauseated by the image of parts of my body being removed. Josh read every relevant medical study he could find online multiple times, learning foreign medical terms and making reasoned conclusions about my prognosis that left him more hopeful. I read one sentence of one study and felt drowsiness setting in, and that was the end of that endeavor to take my medical care into my own hands. Josh puts his faith in science, based on numbers and reason. I put my faith in me and a higher power, based seemingly on nothing tangible, in what some would call complete irrationality.

As irrational as it may seem, my faith comes from my memories, from an understanding of my own history, and to a lesser degree, the history of my parents and those who came before them. My very first memory is of crawling up the narrow staircase of our house in Tam Ky, Vietnam, where there was no railing to protect me from falling onto the dust-covered cement floor. My second memory is of sitting on my grandmother's lap on the Vietnamese fishing boat on the South China Sea, a bare, dim bulb swinging overhead (in my blindness, I could still detect some light and motion) and the mournful prayers of three hundred people begging to reach the safety of the refugee camps in Hong Kong ringing in my ears. I remember a year later trying to fight off the mask that would deliver the general anesthesia in advance of my first sight-giving surgery, at the Jules Stein Eye Institute at UCLA. I remember lugging my large-print book around and all the other kids staring at me like I was a freak. I remember not being able to fill out the answer sheet for the PSATs my sophomore year in high school because the bubbles were too small for me to see them, even with my magnifying glass, and sobbing for the rest of that weekend, feeling the weight of all my limitations. I remember the elation I felt when I told my parents over the phone I had just been accepted into Harvard Law School and how I heard my father clapping with possibly more joy than I felt, like a little boy who had gotten what he wanted for Christmas.

There are so many more memories, both joyful and painful, but I think anyone can understand based on these memories alone why I have faith in myself and some unseen hand. I have felt God's presence more than once in my life, and I have felt his absence. And in those times when God was otherwise occupied, I found, through my shame, frustration, heartache, self-pity, and self-loathing, a strength and resolve that I didn't know I had.

When I woke up at 4:00 A.M. the day after my colonoscopy, the day after we learned that I had colon cancer and before I was transferred to UCLA for the surgery, during what I would call the darkest hours of my life, after I realized that this wasn't a nightmare from which I would awaken, the fear overcame me and I couldn't breathe as I sobbed hysterically into the lonely darkness of that miserable hospital. The future, however long or short, loomed ahead of me, a mass of pure darkness the approximate shape of the mass inside of me. I dug deep then into my past, to find another moment of comparable fear. In truth, there was no fear that I had ever experienced that was comparable to that. But there was one memory that was close, which came during the summer after my first year of law school, when I went to Bangladesh. Although I yearned for what I knew would be an enriching experience, I was terrified. A little Asian girl who can't see very well going alone to one of the poorest countries in the world without any familiarity with the language or culture—it was a bit daunting. Bangladesh, in the days and months before my trip, seemed shrouded in shadows. What if I was mugged or got into a terrible accident or developed dengue fever? I remember acknowledging the fears and doing everything I could within my control to mitigate the risks—I had my mother sew secret pockets for my money and passport into my underwear; I worked out hard so I could be physically strong and fight as fiercely as I could if I were attacked; I bought travel insurance. Then I let everything else go and put faith in myself and a higher power, and I just walked forward, through the fear, into my incredible adventure. Rather than shrouded in shadows, Bangladesh was and is a beautiful place filled with vibrant colors and kind people. My dark prognostications had been wrong.

That night in the hospital room, I willed myself to again acknowledge the fear, told myself to do everything within my power to control my destiny and let everything else go, and then ordered myself to look ahead and walk through the fear once more.

Allende describes her life as a "multilayered and ever-changing fresco that only I can decipher, whose secret is mine alone. The mind selects, enhances, and betrays; happenings fade from memory; people forget one another and, in the end, all that remains is the journey of the soul, those rare moments of spiritual revelation. What actually happened isn't what matters, only the resulting scars and distinguishing marks. My past has little meaning; I can see no order to it, no clarity, purpose, or path, only a blind journey guided by instinct and detours caused by events beyond my control. There was no deliberation on my part, only good intentions and the faint sense of a greater design determining my steps."

Each of us has a story. Each of us has experiences from which we can draw strength and that can serve as the basis of our faith. It is just a matter of whether we are willing to dwell in often unpleasant memories, to extract the lessons of our history, to find the secrets of the journeys of our souls. Just as Allende sought to give the secret of her life story, her past and her memories, to her daughter, I find myself wanting to do so for my daughters.

38

Home

Just after the new year, scans showed that I had failed the clinical trial I had been on at Memorial Sloan Kettering (or more accurately, the trial had failed me). The scans revealed growth in abdominal lymph nodes and two new lesions on my liver (which I suppose is preferable to new lesions *in* my liver). The news was, while not unexpected, still upsetting, because I now have involvement in another vital organ, another way by which the cancer could actually kill me. Will it be my lungs or my liver? There was some shrinkage and some growth in my lungs, so the thoracic tumors were overall unchanged. I lost my hair for that awful trial, suffered unbelievable fatigue, underwent an atrocious lung biopsy, and for what? Absolutely nothing!

Dr. V. offered to put me on Lonsurf, which is standard of care. It is oral chemotherapy that has shown limited effectiveness in a subset of colorectal cancer patients and at best can only offer stability for several months. When I had consulted with Dr. M. at Georgetown in October, he told me he always prescribes Avastin with Lonsurf because they operate on different pathways. Based on his recommendation and the tolerable nature of Avastin, I wanted to do the same. Dr. V. told me Memorial Sloan Kettering doesn't do that. Why? Because that combi-

nation is not indicated, Dr. V. told me (i.e., there are no studies to support the combination, although there are no studies to not support
that combination, either). I left her office, emailed Dr. A.C. while on
the subway, and received a response minutes later, saying that he would
prescribe the Avastin with Lonsurf for me, assuming there was no ob-
jection from the insurance company. He secured both for me in less
than two weeks.

I left home, for college, when I was seventeen years old, and other
than short stints, I never went back. For years, I lived in dorm rooms,
homes of host families abroad, sublets, and apartments with short
leases. I flitted about, going to school, studying abroad, traveling,
working, and then more school, and then more work and more travel.
I craved newness—new places, new people, new challenges. Strangeness was frightening, but mostly it was exciting. I didn't have a home
to call my own, but that didn't matter to me. I was poor most of the
time. The more uncomfortable my habitat the better, because that
meant I was saving money.

Back then, I thought I would live forever, that I was invincible, and
I embraced my freedom with an abandon that belongs only to the
young. I wasn't so different from anyone else in her late teens and
twenties. But age and kids and actually earning a decent living changed
me, and cancer even more so. I have become a creature who yearns for
comfort, for a sense of security, for home. It's obvious in the way I
cried hysterically amid the impersonal unfamiliarity of MSK and how
gratefully I returned to NYU. It's obvious in the way I just want to actually be at home all the time now.

After eight months of construction, a couple more months of
punch list items and hanging things on the wall, and buying a piano
(our last piece of new furniture), the home that Josh and I dared to
dream of in the summer of 2015, despite the ever-present black cancer
cloud, has been realized. I cannot determine what I love most about
our new home: the oak-patterned, gilded wallpaper that accents one
of my bedroom walls; the mantel over the new electric fireplace made
from a piece of reclaimed walnut; the row of custom-built closets with
lights that automatically go on and off with the opening and closing of

the doors; radiant heating in the bathroom floors; or the motorized window treatments. I made all the design decisions—thank you, Josh, for giving me so much latitude—knowing that this place would be the last place I will inhabit and most certainly would be where my family and friends will come see me in my final days and where I will die. I wanted it to be a place of as much luxury and comfort as Josh and I could afford.

Much more important than that, I designed it, knowing that it will be the place in which my children will grow up. I had to think about the adjustable nature of shelving in their closets, the versatility of a bathtub over a shower stall over time, and how the extra room could serve as a playroom now and then one day as a teenage hangout separate and away from the adults. I think of the apartment as a gift to my children, a tangible legacy of a home that I hope they will treasure for many years.

Now, there are many nights when I lie on Mia's or Belle's bed staring up at the princess chandelier that hangs above and I recall all the nights that I lay on my own bed as a little girl and then as an adolescent. Of course, back then my mattress was lumpy and dented, and I stared at a popcorn ceiling and an ugly square overhead light fixture with a giant black screw in the middle. But it was in that childhood bedroom—a room that has long since been demolished together with the rest of the house—that I wondered about my future, about the faceless and nameless man I would one day marry, about what seemed like four long years at a faraway college that loomed ahead. It was there that I dreamed of seeing the world, of traveling, of adventure and romance. I stressed about exams and worried about friendship dramas that I no longer remember. Now I lie on my daughters' beds and wonder what thoughts, fears, and dreams will course through their minds and hearts as they lie in that exact same position. I think to myself, as I stare at these rooms I built just for them, that if I concentrate hard enough, I will leave a bit of me behind in this place, so that when they lie in their beds with exhaustion or anxiety or hope, I will be there to share in those most intimate thoughts and feelings, that a part of my spirit will always be with them, especially in this place. To the extent that a place can convey anything of substance about those who labored to make it, I hope their bedrooms, their bathroom, this entire apartment, their home, will bestow upon them the absolute certainty that their mother loved them so very much.

Home is where I am now. And, in a sense, home is where I will always be, even after I am physically gone from this world.

39

Believe

I love Roger Federer. For those of you who don't know, he is, most would say, the greatest male tennis player of all time (GOAT!). I'm more of a Federer fan than I am a tennis fan. It all started when I met Josh, who was and is a lover of all sports (other than hockey and soccer), but tennis seemed to throw him especially into alternating periods of gut-wrenching anxiety and euphoria, and Roger Federer especially so. He would watch Wimbledon or the Australian Open matches on tape delay and absolutely despair when Federer dropped a set. I didn't know anything about Federer back then and thought Josh was just crazy; how stupid to care so much about two men hitting a tiny ball back and forth. I'd secretly go online and find out Federer had won the match—Josh hates watching sports with anyone who already knows the outcome—and then tell him lovingly, "It's going to be okay, honey." Back then, Federer was in his prime and racking up Grand Slam titles at an astounding pace as he sought to surpass Pete Sampras's Grand Slam record of fourteen. Josh, as do most people, loves to watch dominance, to marvel at human physical excellence, and Roger Federer was a prime example of the incredible feats that the human body is capable of. My feigned interest in basketball and football disappeared after we got engaged and then married, but my love for Federer persisted.

After our wedding, in the fall of 2007, Federer's physical decline began. Josh and I would watch matches together with greater stress as the odds of his victory decreased with the passing of the months and years. When Federer sought to tie Pete Sampras's record at the 2009 Australian Open, we got up at 3:00 A.M. to watch the finals against Federer's archrival, Rafael Nadal, the other arguable GOAT. It was a disastrous match for Federer; he crumbled under the pressure of history. Our household of two was in mourning that day. And yet, I'm pretty sure that Mia was conceived that night—as they say, out of the ashes of defeat . . .

When I was seven months pregnant with Mia, we forked over the big bucks to go see Federer play in the fourth round at the U.S. Open on Labor Day. We sat in the front row, right behind the service line. You could see us on TV all day long. I was in ecstasy to have my tennis God so close.

Federer would make it to the finals of that U.S. Open, but he would lose to Argentinian Juan Martín del Potro. Josh went to the finals while I stayed home to watch. He would call me during the commercial breaks to give me his impressions from the court. I would tell him what John McEnroe was saying on TV. I had become as crazy as he.

Federer, however, would go on to win more slams. The last, number 17, was the 2012 Wimbledon championship. The morning of my colonoscopy on July 7, 2013, the day I was diagnosed with colon cancer, Novak Djokovic lost the Wimbledon final to the hated Andy Murray; Federer had been eliminated in an earlier round. How apropos. Josh had watched the match early that morning, before he came to the hospital to be with me as I was wheeled away. We were in California, which meant even more of a time difference. Wimbledon barely registered to me that year.

The following year, Federer again made it to the Wimbledon finals. As I had so many times before, I watched in my apartment, glued to the TV and yet throwing a blanket over my head during the high-pressure moments. Even though I knew it was ludicrous, I told myself that if Roger Federer could win another slam despite becoming an old man in tennis terms, then I could beat cancer. Of course, at that point, my cancer had not metastasized to my lungs. Federer lost in a five-setter to Djokovic. I was devastated, for him, but mostly for myself.

In the years that followed, Federer didn't win. He made it deep into many Grand Slam tournaments, quarters and semis but no finals. Injuries began to plague him as he moved into his mid-thirties. I stopped watching. I told Josh it was game over for our beloved Federer, that it was time for him to retire with grace, that I didn't want him to be humiliated by these younger guys. Josh never gave up on him, though. Never. Josh believed as I have never seen anyone believe. He kept telling me that as long as Fed could go deep into a Grand Slam tournament, he still had a chance.

Federer cut his 2016 season short by six months to recover from knee surgery. No one, including him, was expecting much at the Australian Open, the first Grand Slam of the year. Even so, he looked good in the rounds leading up to the finals. I still wasn't watching. Josh questioned whether Federer should even strive to make the finals because it was looking more and more likely that he would meet Nadal, at whose hands he had suffered so much defeat, there; Nadal had long ago gotten into Federer's head. Could Fed handle yet another defeat? Could *we*? I told Josh I didn't think I could bear to watch another Federer defeat, and to Nadal no less. It would simply crush me. Josh got up early to watch the finals on tape delay, with me rising soon thereafter (after I had, of course, looked online to see that he had been broken early in the fifth set—not good at all; most assuredly he was on his way to losing). But I got up anyhow to support my devoted husband, with the slimmest bit of hope in the final outcome. Josh confiscated my phone when he saw me trying to sneak another look at a live update. So I really had no idea what was about to happen.

Somehow, some way, with the momentum against him, Federer dug deep and held serve and proceeded to break Nadal to level the set, held his own serve easily again, and then broke Nadal again. He won the match soundly shortly thereafter. Josh and I, our hearts racing, were jumping up and down, dancing for joy, hugging, kissing, high-fiving. The kids would definitely have thought we were certifiably crazy, but we had locked them in our bedroom at the far end of the apartment and turned on nonstop *Monster High*. In his postmatch interviews, Federer spoke of how sweet this victory was, given that it had taken him so long, given how hard he had worked, given his age, given all the naysayers.

Josh never stopped believing in Federer. He has never stopped believing in me, either, never. Even when I've said that it's game over for me, that I am dying. I told him that this past birthday would be my last. My emphatic statements and the disheartening scan results no doubt have made him question his own belief, but he still held firm. I told him he was delusional, that he just couldn't accept my death, that he had to tell himself I still had a chance for his own sanity. He would look at my skin and watch how I move about and he would say, You're not dying. He would say, As long as you are still playing, you still have a chance.

Federer won, and I felt like that was a sign in late January, that I had to actually start listening to my husband. Horror of horrors! But what else was I supposed to do exactly?

40

Pain

For a week, I've been trying to write, but nothing comes out. Nothing coherent. Nothing good. I am in chaos, and so there can be no good writing under the circumstances.

I have been unable to persuade Dr. Y., the radiation oncologist, to move up radiation treatment on my spine. He didn't perceive any immediate danger; he said the tumor seemed to be growing into my bone, rather than toward my spinal cord. I suppose he was right, since I made it to the radiation treatment on June 5 without becoming paralyzed beforehand. In fact, the pain seemed to ease in the interim. I was shocked and attributed it to my conscious effort to sleep with proper alignment. I had three radiation treatments on consecutive days. The treatments themselves were uneventful, quick and easy enough. It was the aftereffects I hadn't quite expected. Pain. Excruciating, throbbing pain in my upper right back, the kind of pain that had me sitting up at night, desperate to rip that part of my body out. I turned to oxycodone, which relieved the pain but had me feeling washed out the next day, very sleep-deprived, nauseated and vomiting multiple times in twelve hours. Apparently, it is normal for the pain to get worse before it gets better after radiation. Of course, no one told me this. I thought many times that if I couldn't manage the pain, I would have to go to the ER—that's how bad it was. Fortunately, the pain did get better after almost a week and is now nearly entirely gone.

But now I have pain elsewhere. Pain in my left butt and leg that has steadily worsened over the last few weeks. I'm convinced I have a new met in my lumbar spine.

I've been experiencing random vaginal bleeding as well—sorry if that's too much information, but why should I hide that since I talk about everything else? Of course, I'm worried it is a second primary cancer. It took weeks to get an appointment with a gynecological oncologist at MSK, who took some Pap smears and did a uterine biopsy. While she couldn't say for sure until the results were back, she thought my bleeding issues were more likely caused by the location of metastases from the colon cancer. I don't know what would happen if I had a second primary cancer. The idea of it seems unbearable to contemplate, but in truth, everything I've endured during these past four years at one point seemed unbearable to contemplate.

Finally, the tumor next to my belly button has been bothering me a lot again. I can literally feel it now, probably because of my drastic weight loss. The current study drugs robbed me of the ability to taste for many weeks, which caused me to lose a lot of weight, since I lost interest in food and ate solely to not be hungry. I can taste now, although nothing tastes right, so my appetite is still not where it once was. Additionally, the vomiting from the opiates hasn't helped.

Back to the tumor. I play with it, rubbing it, imagining it, measuring it. I use my thumb and forefinger to determine its length and then hold those fingers up against a ruler—roughly two centimeters, just as the last scan report said. I touch it, caress it, worship it, almost as if it were a rabbit's foot, a manifestation of God, to whom I can pray for salvation. Sometimes it feels like it's answering my prayers, like it's calmed down, shrinking even. Sometimes it feels enraged, big and furious at me for trying to sway its will. In the end, it controls my mood. When it is calm, I am calm (optimistic even). When it's angry, I am angry (and scared and sad). But more important, I know it controls me and whether and when I live and die.

I scheduled another round of scans for the middle of June. The scans will likely be very bad if pain and just my general physical well-being are gauges. I'm trying to prepare myself for the worst. But I don't know how to. I don't know what the next steps would be, if there would be next steps for me. Instead, I struggle with being okay with dying. I tell myself that I've lived a good life. I tell myself that I am not afraid of dying, that I am so tired and in so much pain, I want to die at this point. Most of the time this is true, but I am not fully there yet. I haven't found the peace I so desperately want, the kind of peace in which I would be okay with a bad scan, knowing that death is coming that much sooner. Peace is all I really want. The question is, How do I find it?

41

Death, Part Two

I was Daddy's little girl, his favorite, his precious one, his gold nugget. He would tell anyone and everyone exactly that, in Vietnamese or Chinese. It was embarrassing, especially in those teenage years, but I loved him, too, even if he was often too nosy and annoying in so many other ways. Perhaps it was because I was the child most like him, inquisitive and interested in the world and its people. Perhaps in me he saw all his own potential and dreams never realized—the intellectual, the fearless world traveler, the moneymaking professional. In him, I saw a man who loved me beyond measure, who would spend hours in traffic driving me to and from the airport, high school competitions, study group sessions, and the orthodontist, who believed that I could walk on the moon if I so chose. Sometimes, I felt somewhat bad for my older brother and sister. He loved them, too, of course, but it just wasn't the same. (It was widely known, however, that my brother was my mother's favorite and my sister was my grandmother and the uncles' favorite, so I didn't feel too bad.) During one of our many car rides together, I asked my father, "Don't you think that it is not right for you to love me more than Older Brother and Older Sister?" He took his right hand off the steering wheel and held it out to me, its fingers stretched. "Look at my hand," he ordered. "You see my fingers?

Are they even? No. It isn't possible to love your children the same."
And that was that. My father, the sage Chinese philosopher, had
spoken.

Anyhow, knowing that he loved me as much as he did, I felt incredibly sorry for him as he stood helplessly by when I left for college three
thousand miles away from home and then on my various adventures
to far-flung places, the kinds of impoverished places that we had risked
our lives to escape. He was and is a worrier. He would sit morosely
watching me, shoulders drooped, as I packed for my next adventure,
wringing his hands and running his fingers through his virtually non-
existent hair. Sure, I was nervous about my travels, somewhat afraid of
what I might encounter, but mostly I was excited and enthralled by the
promise and possibility of newness and all the things to be seen and
experienced. I was off to have fun, to grow and learn, to be changed
and challenged; my father would be left behind at home, worrying.
His life centered on me, and that center was leaving. I swore then that
I never wanted to be the one left behind, even if I were to have my own
children, that I was and would forever be an intrepid traveler and ad-
venturer.

It seems that with the latest bad scan results, I will continue to
make good on that promise I made myself so long ago. I will be the
one to die young. I will be the first among so many family and friends
to embark on the greatest adventure of all, the one that involves traveling beyond this life into the next. Were the choice mine, I would stay
longer, to watch my children grow up and to age with my husband, to
bury my parents, to see more of this life that I have loved so much. But
the choice is not mine. It has never been mine.

I am busily packing my bags now. I am making my lists, leaving my
instructions, putting in place my final estate-planning documents. I am
making my final memories, saying my goodbyes, telling everyone I
love them, writing my last words. I am noting not just all the people I
will miss but also the things of life I will miss. I will miss the simple
ritual of loading and unloading the dishwasher. I will miss the smooth
patina of my cast-iron skillet, brought on by cooking countless meals.
I will miss making Costco runs. I will miss watching TV with Josh. I

will miss taking my kids to school. I will miss this life so very much. They say that youth is wasted on the young. Now, as I approach my final days, I realize that health is wasted on the healthy, and life is wasted on the living. I never understood that until now, as I prepare in earnest to leave this life.

Sleep no longer matters. I tell myself as I race against time to make the flight, before the pain settles in, before my mind becomes addled by opiates, that there will be time enough to sleep later. Sadly, this time it's not just my father who sits helplessly by; it's also Josh and my children, my mother and siblings, cousins and so many friends. I'm sorry for that. I'm sorry to leave it to others to pick up the pieces. It is a selfish act, perhaps unknowingly brought on by a selfish promise I made so long ago. But believe me when I say that this is not of my conscious choosing.

I know that soon I will stand on the brink of something extraordinary, something greater than the human mind can understand. I have far greater faith in the belief that there is more than this life than I do in a God. I know with every fiber of my being that there is an afterlife. I keep thinking about all the people I have met who have died since my diagnosis four years ago—Debbie, Carlyle, Rachel, Colleen, Chris, Jane, and so many more—and I realize that they taught me how to die, that I will follow in their footsteps, that they and others in my family wait to greet me and help me make the transition. And that makes me happy. When I was pregnant with Mia and nervous about giving birth, I consoled myself with the thought that billions of women have done exactly the same thing for millennia, and so there should be no reason why I couldn't do it and do it well. Similarly, I think now of all these people I know who have died and the billions of people who have died over the millennia, and there is no reason why I cannot also embark on this rite of passage and do it well.

It is my absolute goal to die well, to die at peace, without regret for the life I have lived, proud and satisfied. Why do we always assume that the ideal life is a long one? Why do we assume that it is so awful to die young? Could it be that the ones who die young are better off? Could it be that death offers greater wisdom and joy than this life and those who die young are indeed lucky in their ability to attain those gifts sooner? Perhaps these are simply the musings of a person desperately trying to come to terms with her own early death. And yet, I can assure you that I feel no desperation (other than the desperation to finish all the preparations before it's too late), that if anything I feel almost total and complete peace.

I do not know if peace comes to all or just to those who seek it, to those who rage or to those who surrender, but over the months of 2017, peace came to me.

42

Preparing

Mia is in third grade, and Belle is in first grade. As school started, parents came together and engaged in some version of the game of one-upmanship, as each tried to "one-up" the others, to wear the cloak for Best and Coolest Summer. Trips to France, Spain, Italy, *blah, blah, blah*. Of course, I played the game, too. A part of me needed to play, to feel like despite everything, I could still give my children a semblance of a normal childhood and a summer that could rival anyone's. "Mia and Belle went to South Carolina to see their grandparents, which put them in the path of the total solar eclipse. They loved it. They'll never forget the experience," I bragged. Even as I said the words, I wondered why I bother at this stage of my life, why I engage in the stupid, vapid games, why any of it matters at all.

I should have just opened my mouth and stunned them with the truth: "The girls went to South Carolina to see their grandparents and to see the total solar eclipse, but I agonized over whether to allow them to go because I was afraid of losing time with them while they were away for twelve days, or worse yet, that I would die while they were gone. But I realized I had to let them go because that is a necessary part of preparing to die, and that's what I did this summer— prepare to die. And they may not have been aware of it, but they were also preparing for me to die, to let me go, to start forging their own way in this world without their mother. That's what our family did this summer. So, why don't you top that?"

Oh, how I would have loved to see the looks on their faces if I had said all that. How I would have loved to see the shock when hearing complete, absolute, and uncomfortable truth.

The scans in late June that marked the beginning of the children's summer break also marked the true beginning of the end of my life. I knew it. For two months, this most promising of clinical trials, this trial for which Phase I data had been presented at the annual meeting of clinical oncologists earlier that month (something reserved for only the most exciting of early research findings), had worked. It had shrunk the tumors, even dramatically, it seemed. I've often observed how metastatic cancer and the bodies it inhabits seem to find an equilibrium for a time, some balance between stability or slow progression and treatment, where both live in a relatively peaceful coexistence based on a mutual agreement not to bother each other. But then I bothered the cancer, and it got really, really mad. *How dare you fuck with me?* it raged. And in response to my daring to attack it, it grew and grew and grew and continues to grow. I had disturbed the beast, and I have paid the price. The met next to my belly button now feels like a golf ball, with more masses nearby. The mets in my pelvis are growing quickly as well, and at some point I expect they will block my digestive tract so that I will no longer be able to eat, at which point I will consider the viability and desirability of being fed artificially. But death comes only when there is failure of a vital organ. For now, my lungs and liver are functioning properly, although I have no idea for how long that will be true. Based on my observations, near the end, cancer becomes even more aggressive, growing at an even faster rate, until it consumes the body it depends on for life. How stupid cancer is, indeed. If only I could negotiate a truce. But despite how it may seem, cancer is not a sentient being with intelligence or reason.

Grieving is a necessary part of preparation, too, so that's what I did this summer—grieve. After those scan results, I grieved for the life that will never be, the vacation to Tahiti with Josh that will remain a dream, the African safari with the girls that will be without me, the trip to Vietnam to show the girls where their mother was born with my sister instead of me. I grieved and grieve for my declining body, for the fact that running next door to Target or the bank is now a monumental endeavor, for my atrophying muscles and sagging skin, for the fear of being too far from home and a bed or a couch, for the body that cares not at all about what others may think as it needs to squat on the side-walk when no bench is in sight so the abdominal pain might ease. Is this what it's like to age, but at high speed, I often wonder.

I summoned my parents to me. I wanted my mother to make my favorite soups and my father to buy me my favorite Chinese pastries. I hesitated at first, because I thought it would be too difficult to watch my parents absorb the fact of my dying. There can be nothing more cruel than watching your own child die. I understand that, now that I am a mother. But my sister insisted that it would be better for us to all grieve together than apart, that they would feel better being with me than not with me. So my siblings and I purchased one-way tickets for them, their stay achingly indefinite. For a while, my mother drove me nuts as she insisted on my drinking and eating weird Chinese medicine crap that I don't believe in and balked at my father's purchase of all the unhealthy Chinese pastries I wanted to eat. I told her I could now eat whatever the fuck I wanted, and my father would bark some words at her, effectively telling her to shut up. Every night, when my parents returned to my sister's apartment, my sister and my father would tell my mother to leave me alone, let me enjoy what time there was left for me, and trust that I knew what I wanted for myself. At one point, her pestering got so bad I threatened to throw her out of my apartment and send her back to Los Angeles. After that, she stopped.

I spent my summer saying goodbye. I summoned my brother. I wanted him to come sharpen my knives and oil my cutting board and change the water filters under the kitchen sink. I wanted us to make one last trip to Costco together because that's what Chinese siblings who love deals do together. My brother stayed for only a weekend in late July. The night before he was to leave, the five of us—my parents, my sister, my brother, and I—sat in my dining room, not saying much, knowing that it would be the last time we would really be together, that the next time my brother flew the thousands of miles to New York I would be within days or hours of death. Mau and I kept peppering my sister with instructions on how to be a surrogate mother, but it was what was unsaid that resonated in that room. The phones and cameras came out as we silently acknowledged to one another how precious and fleeting these moments were. For forty-one years, it had been the five of us. This was my family, even though we kids had grown up and gone on to have our own lives and families. This was still my family, our family. And I knew that going forward, in future family photographs, there would be a glaring absence, a heartbreaking hole that could never be filled. My parents will never have another daughter, and my siblings will never have another sister. Forty-one years together finished in that room on that night.

I spent my summer planning. I bought a new mattress for Mia because the old one was lumpy, and if I didn't do it, it might never get done and Mia would be stuck sleeping on an uncomfortable bed for God knows how long. I found the girls a child psychologist. I found a chef to prepare meals for the girls and Josh. I started the process of finding the girls a high school or college student who will attend music lessons with them and oversee their practices. I will soon check this off my list. I wouldn't be a true Chinese tiger mom if I didn't safeguard their musical progress.

I bought my burial plot. I will be buried at Green-Wood, a historic and unexpectedly beautiful cemetery in the heart of Brooklyn, where some pretty famous people are buried. I'm told a plot is hard to come by, but I got lucky. For four years I had planned on cremation. I used to tell Josh that I wanted my body to burn, that I wanted the cancer to burn, that it deserved nothing less. But then when the time came to make the final arrangements, I realized that I could not abide the idea of burning my own body, that the desire to burn my body and eviscerate the cancer came from a place of such hatred and rage that I could not allow that to be the final message of my body. As much as I hate the cancer, for thirty-seven years my body served me well. It took me all over the world and gave me two beautiful little girls. I could not let the cancer destroy all the goodness that had once been. Then there's the fact that I've always hated fire. I don't even like to light a match.

The idea of my body being taken to a cold and institutional cremato-rium seemed even more repulsive. Plus, Josh wants to have a place to go to visit me. He wants to have a place to bring the girls to visit me. He wants to be able to lie at rest next to me. As it turned out, I want what Josh wants.

But mostly, I spent the summer thinking about how I want to live and spend my remaining months in this life.

I went to the Galápagos Islands two summers ago. It was Josh and me and thirty other passengers on a boat that went from island to is-land to see all kinds of crazy birds with blue webbed feet and red bal-loon chests that puffed out like gigantic hearts, and meandering hundred-year-old giant tortoises, and sea lions that swam right along-side as you snorkeled (the ocean's version of puppy dogs). On one is-land we saw the skeleton of a long-dead seal that had no doubt been picked away by scavengers, not a hundred feet away from a very much alive mother seal and her cubs. It was the kind of remote place where you knew you were witnessing life's primordial roots, Mother Nature at its most primal, millions of years of untamed life undisturbed by human activity; after all, this was where Charles Darwin first gave breath to his theories of survival of the fittest and evolution.

One night after dinner on the boat, someone spotted a shark glid-ing through the waters. The boat came to a standstill so we could ob-serve the shark. The lights from the boat cast a faint glint on the shark's slippery body. Soon, we realized that the shark was in fact in pursuit of a fish, a fly fish, I think it was called. The fish, desperate to get away, literally flew out of the water and plopped right in the middle of the deck and started flopping around as if in its panic it would find a way to save its own life. What should we do? We could not save the fish. I suppose we could have moved the boat to another position and then thrown the fish back into the water. But surely, the shark or another predator would have found him in his compromised state. Eventually, one of our guides threw the fish back into the dark ocean, where he was swallowed whole by the shark and the waters soon returned to their usual calm.

I've thought about that fish often since. I know that the primordial instincts in him to survive, to save himself, lie within me, too. I know the base desperation he felt. I feel that desperate panic each time I notice my tumors growing again. I've seen the same instincts in others facing death. There was that guy who talked about potential clinical trials even as his lungs were about to be drained; he died five days later in the hospital. (In case you were wondering, when tubes need to be inserted to remove unwanted fluid, it is generally a sign that the end is near and that one is not healthy enough for a clinical trial.) Then there are the people in support groups who dole out the stupidest and most thoughtless advice, advice that is reflective of that same base desperate instinct to survive at all cost. To a patient considering stopping all treatments and going into hospice, they often say, "You have to keep going. Giving up is not an option." One mother, who has since died, after being told by her doctor that she had eighteen months (she died much sooner), said, "Dying is not an option." I thought to myself then, *Really?* And then I wondered, as her death became evident even to her, What did she think? Did she continue to think death was not an option? In fact and in reality, death is truly what is inevitable and life is the option.

These statements come from the same group of people who spew asinine assertions about how there is always hope, because look at their situations when they had limited cancer and they made it. But where's the hope for me and others like me? Where's the hope for my friend Amy, who just died one year after diagnosis, leaving behind a two-year-old daughter? Where's the hope for the millions who have died from cancer?

At some point, the reality and inevitability of death must be acknowledged and accepted. People who make such thoughtless statements when faced with death allow their baser instincts to govern; they choose to be more like primordial fish than evolved human beings. These are the people who are so afraid of death they cannot approach it with the dignity and grace that befit an evolved soul.

I may have some of the instincts of that fish, but I am not that fish. We, as human beings, are not that fish. We are evolved. We have reason. We are capable of a thoughtful and meaningful existence that transcends our primal roots, and that is what I aspire to, and I daresay it is what every human being should aspire to. Our best humanity means being able to control our baser instincts, to squelch the panic and fear, to overcome with reason and intellect and compassion and honesty and faith and love.

What also distinguishes us from primordial fish is our ability to choose our fate. Self-will and self-determination are fundamental elements of what it means to be human, elements of ourselves that should be cherished and celebrated. Within certain confines, and even as there is so much beyond our control, you and I get to choose our destinies. And when I, or anyone else, am told that I don't have an option, that I must act based on some mindless instinct, it takes away from the beauty of my humanity and my individual choice. This applies to any life context, not just cancer. For the person who battles depression and struggles to get up every morning but does so anyhow, I applaud that choice. For the person who battles depression and wants to commit suicide and take his life into his own hands in an exercise of his self-determination, I applaud that choice, too, so long as it is made with cogency. Similarly, for the person who with thought and clarity chooses hospice over more treatment and more clinical trials, or vice versa, I applaud you. I celebrate you. Bravo!

Whatever the world or my children may think of me after I am gone, I hope that at the very least no one will think of me as a thoughtless, mindless person, desperate to stay alive. I hope the world knows that I approached my death with clarity, that I made my decisions not out of panic but with reason, intellect, compassion, honesty, and love, from the best parts of my humanity. At least, this is my goal.

Within a week of receiving my scan results, I had an appointment at Mount Sinai to discuss the results of the fruit fly study in which I have been participating. For eighteen months, researchers at Mount Sinai had worked on creating fruit fly avatars containing my tumors from the original primary colon tumor. They had identified one potential drug combination. Out of a library of twelve hundred FDA-approved drugs, one combination, which consisted of two drugs, had resulted in my fruit flies still living. The test was not a measure of tumor shrinkage within the fruit flies; rather, it was simply a question of whether the fruit flies were still standing when everything was said and done. The flies survived the cancer only with this drug combination. One drug the insurance company would easily approve. The other is a melanoma drug, not approved for colorectal cancer, and therefore the insurance would not pay for it. The pharmaceutical company also refused to give me the drug because I didn't meet their rather stringent income limitations. I did find a specialty mail-order pharmacy that would provide me the drug at a cost of seven thousand dollars a month. Theoretically, I could pay for the drug for two months, and if the scans showed the drug combination was working, I would have an argument with the insurance company for reimbursement.

In the big scheme of things, seven thousand dollars a month is not a huge amount of money for me and Josh, and I could have comfortably spent that sum for a couple months. But I was less than impressed with the fact that the trial had not found a way to cover the cost of the drug when applied to patients; to me, that did not say much about the researchers' faith in their findings. Second, I continued to be skeptical about whether results in fruit flies would be effectively replicated in human beings; it is hard enough to reproduce mice results in humans, and these are two mammals with much more similar biologies. Plus, the testing had been performed on my primary tumor, which most certainly is not an accurate biological representation of my metastasized cancer. Third, there was the time and energy to be expended with this or any other trial. I have participated in three experimental treatments, two of them clinical trials. I am well aware of the extensive testing required, and at this point, I don't have much time or energy to spare on something with a 99.9 percent chance of failure. I'd much rather be at home with my children or hanging out with friends or writing or even lounging on my couch watching TV.

I am tired.

Memorial Sloan Kettering offered me a spot in an immunotherapy trial. It seemed decent, but they withdrew the spot after I signed the consent. Yale said I was more than healthy enough for another clinical trial, but they didn't have a spot in the trial I wanted. Anyway, I wouldn't have wanted to spend the time traveling two hours each way to New Haven. At some point, the clinical trials these renowned institutions throw at you don't seem all that different from the green-sludge swamp water from Mexico I swore I would never drink. Acts of desperation made barely palatable by a thin veneer of science performed on mice— that's all clinical trials are. Call me a little jaded by my experiences. So I said no to the clinical trials and decided to recycle FOLFOX, my first chemotherapy combination, at a reduced dose. It seemed like the treatment with the best odds of working, something I could point to to show the girls that their mother didn't completely give up at the end. I've had three treatments. At this point, I don't need scans to tell me if a treatment is working. I can feel the cancer growing. It's not working. I will stop soon, and then it will be time for hospice. Unless, of course, my baser instincts kick in despite my best intentions.

I've always known that I would bring in hospice early, that I wanted the hospice people to get to know me and my family. I've always wanted to die at home and not in the hospital. And in order to ensure that, hospice must be brought onboard early enough. Too many times, I've heard of patients going to the hospital to deal with symptoms and then not being able to get out. It can be difficult to escape the vortex of cascading complications that can arise from end-stage cancer and the interventions performed in hospitals. I also see families asking for pri-vacy in the end as they close ranks around the dying. I think this in large part stems from a culture that is terrified of dying and death, a culture that likes to hide or run in shame from death and pretend until the very end like it isn't happening and isn't real. I have always known that for me, this is not the right choice. I love people. I love life. I want to be surrounded by both as I bid my final farewell. To the extent I can exert control, I will die on my terms. That I have promised myself. I want my children to be with me. I want my home to be filled with family and friends and laughter and tears and stories and food, the very best parts of life. I want my children to learn by the example of my death not to be afraid of death, to understand it as simply a part of life. I want them to see how loved their mother was and that, by extension, they are safe and loved. I know a death that is at once lively and peace-ful and filled with love will be one of the greatest gifts I can give them. For four years, I've been planning my death, and now I finally get to execute my plan.

43

Love

Dear Josh,

Sometimes, I can feel the weight of your stare as I feign sleep in those torturous minutes before I fully awaken. Your grip on my hand has tightened; that's what probably woke me in the first instance. I can feel your love. I can feel you trying desperately to save the image of my face in some special place that might be immune to the amnesiac effects of time. I can feel your fear as you unwillingly envision a life without me—how will you comfort the girls like I can; how will you plan the birthday parties and arrange the girls' schedules; how will you fix all the things that break in our home; how will you do all this while still working your demanding job and maintaining the stellar course of your career? In turn, in my own mind's eye, I can see you cleaning out our closets and bathroom drawers to dispose of all my things. I can see you bringing flowers to my grave. I can see you watching what were once "our" favorite TV shows after the girls have gone to bed, in the dark, alone, the television casting its eerie blue light on your face, which seems to be permanently sculpted in sadness. My heart aches for you, but I don't know how to help you. Beyond solving all the logistical problems caused by my death, what can I say or do to alleviate the pain, to make losing me easier for you, if that is even possible? Just as I felt compelled to write the girls a letter, I feel a compulsion to do the same for you in an attempt to help, for to not do so would be a great failure by me as your wife.

When I hug you now, when I scratch your head, when I lie in the crook of your arm, I feel distinctly the finitude of our time together in this life. I try so hard to feel and remember everything I can in a single touch, every pore in my body and soul open to you and you alone, as if I can somehow brand your skin, your hair, your very essence into my soul, so I can take you with me when I leave this world. Does it help you to know this? Understand, Josh, that until I met you, at age thirty, it felt like I had been waiting my whole life for you. Does it help you to know this, too? I've always believed in soul mates, in that one person (or maybe two people) who would effortlessly and seamlessly slip into my life and heart as if he had always been there. At ages ten and twelve and fourteen and sixteen and eighteen, I would lie awake at night, wondering where you were at that very moment, the boy who would one day be the man who would be the love of my life, my Mr. Darcy, my tall, dark, and handsome. What can I say? I've always been a hopeless romantic.

The truth is that nothing I say or do will help you as much as time. Time, that undefinable thing that marks the passing of the seconds, minutes, hours, days, weeks, months, years, and decades; that thing that seems to stretch often agonizingly into eternity and yet is also cruelly gone too quickly; that thing that waits and hurries for, and otherwise spares, nothing and no one; that thing that makes us forget, or at the very least blunts, the good and the bad. Remember how Mia was a day overdue, and you, impatient, were freaking out and demanded that I get induced (which I ignored)? Now she's about to turn eight. In the interim, our faces have aged, imperceptibly in the day-to-day but oh so noticeably when we look back at different moments, as recorded by the photos that do not lie about the passage of time. Time has made you and me forget almost every detail of the night we walked across the Brooklyn Bridge, the night we started to fall in love with one another. Was it fifty-eight or sixty degrees? Was it windy as we looked upon the millions of sparkling lights that constitute the Manhattan skyline? What were you wearing?

Time has robbed our minds of those many beautiful and rich de-tails, and for better or worse, it has also robbed us of that unique eu-phoria of falling in love. The intense excitement and anxiety of falling in love are only memories now, impersonal almost, as if it all happened to somebody else. Sometimes, I wish I could relive those moments, just push a button and for a few glorious minutes travel back in time and be that young, ecstatic woman falling in love with the man of her dreams all over again. But the laws of existence don't allow that. By the same token, I don't remember the innumerable fights we've had, ei-ther, not even the worst ones, in which we threatened divorce. I don't remember what they were about. I know there were occasions when I was so angry I wanted to smack you in the face, but I can't make my-self feel that rage now. Time cares not that you are the man of my dreams, nor does it care about the most egregious wrongs we have committed against one another; it cares not whether the experiences and emotions were wanted or unwanted, loved or hated; it does not discriminate. Eventually, time dulls everything. It removes the inten-sity of the purest of joys and the hottest of rages and, yes, even the most heartbreaking of sorrows.

I remember when my grandmother died, when I was twenty; it was the most painful experience of my young life. I remember crying on the flight back to school. I remember crying through my midterms. My family and I (when I was in town) used to go visit her grave site all the time. She who had been the center of our family was sorely missed. But over the years, the visits became less frequent. Weekly visits be-came monthly and then only on holidays and then annually and then not at all. I haven't been to her grave site in fifteen years. My life and everyone else's life continued. We all grew older. We got married. We had our own children. We went on with the business of living.

One day soon, my whole existence, everything that I am and have been to you, will be memory, growing more distant with the passing of each day. One day, you'll wake up and you won't remember my face easily anymore. You won't remember my smell anymore. You won't remember if I liked chocolate ice cream or not. You won't remember so many things that you might have once thought you could never forget. Or maybe you failed to think of me for one hour or two or three, or for a day. You may even stop visiting me at my grave site with any regularity. I want you to know that that is okay, that that is how it should be, that that is what I want it to be.

Time's amnesiac power is necessary and healthy, for it encourages life and living, allowing room for new experiences and new emotions, which come with engaging in the present and being vested in the future, and places our memories where they should be—in the past, to be accessed when we need and want them. And perhaps most important and relevant to you, time allows for the gaping wounds of the past to close so that we can move forward, so that even the most painful experiences can be remembered with some objectivity, from which we can learn and grow. I want you to go on living, Josh. I want you to obsess about sports. I want you to dine in fine restaurants. I want you to travel the world. I want you to raise our children to the best of your ability, which will require you to be so very present and focused on the here and now.

In the ultimate act of living, I even want you to love again. As hard as that is for me to say, I really do.

We've spent much time over the last four years talking about the Slutty Second Wife, a name I gave the woman who would replace me within days of my diagnosis. Actually, I have been the one talking about her, while you just rolled your eyes. And I wouldn't call it talking; it was more like railing, threatening, and ranting. There are women who write letters to their replacements on their deathbeds, wishing them well, but I'm sorry—I can't. I'm not that generous.

I worry that she will be a gold digger, preying on you in your vulnerable state. I worry that she will be like Cinderella's evil stepmother. I worry that she will seek to destroy all traces of me from your and the girls' lives. I fear that she will not prioritize the girls spending time in Los Angeles so that they can continue their relationship with my family, that she will not care about preserving my legacy. I fear that she will brainwash you, and in the stress and business of life, you will forget what was important to me and all the promises you made me to honor my wishes for the girls. Will she completely redesign this apartment to erase as much of me as she can from the home that I built for you and the girls? Or worse yet, will she force you to sell this apartment, which

I created for you and the girls to enjoy for years to come? As you know, I have hundreds of worries like these. You tell me to have faith in you. You tell me to trust in your ability to make the right decisions. But it's hard for me.

Remember the big argument we had about how much time would have to elapse before you could appropriately start dating, get engaged, get married? You googled and recited to me statistics, percentages, about how soon after a spouse's death the surviving spouse engages in a sexual encounter, in a serious relationship, marriage. There were dramatic differences between widows and widowers, with the widowers doing all of the above much sooner than the widows. For example, 7 percent of widows engaged in a sexual encounter within one year of their spouses' death, whereas 51 percent of widowers did the same. I was horrified and disgusted. Men are inherently so weak and incapable of caring for themselves and being alone. You talked about being engaged a year after I died, married after two at the latest. I was upset, furious at you. Are you so weak and pathetic?

Granted, you've had a long time to prepare for my death. It's not as if my death will be a surprise. But even so, instinctively, I felt like there should be some minimal amount of time to show due respect to me. But how much is the right amount of time?

I have thought about that question a lot. And here's my answer, which I'm going to give you in a roundabout manner, by way of stories.

As I said before, I've always been a hopeless romantic. I suppose it was a reaction to the complete absence of romance in my childhood (except, of course, for what I saw on the screen and read in the romance novels devoured in secret, the ones my father forbade me from reading). Pragmatism was the guiding principle of love and marriage in my immigrant household. Have you ever seen my parents kiss, even on the cheek? Exactly. Neither have I. I can count on one hand the number of times I've seen them even touch one another with any kind of affection. I never saw that between my grandparents, my father's parents, the ones I grew up around. Romantic love was simply not a part of my family tradition.

My grandparents' marriage was arranged when they were still children, despite the fact that they lived in different countries. My grandmother was from a little village in Hainan, a lush island off the coast of southern China. My grandfather's parents had also been born in Hainan, but he himself had been born in Vietnam after his parents immigrated there to start what would become a successful business in trading spices and other valuable commodities, like elephant tusks and rhino horns. The families knew and liked each other. My grandfather's family was well off; my grandmother was young, strong, and healthy. At fourteen, she was plucked from everything and everyone she had ever known and taken to Vietnam on a multiweek boat journey by a stranger, her future husband's maternal grandfather. There, she had to learn a new language and a new way of life that revolved around commerce, and not farming or the land. There, she resentfully did as her domineering mother-in-law commanded while my great-grandmother spent most days gambling. There, she cared for her boy-husband and his seven younger brothers and sisters, even breast-feeding his youngest brother as she breast-fed her own firstborn son. My grandmother cooked, cleaned, sewed, and even massaged the stubs that were my great-grandmother's feet; Great-Grandmother grew up in an era when bound feet no bigger than three inches were a mark of erotic beauty, and so she must have deplored my grandmother's grotesquely large feet. My grandmother was effectively a servant in her own home, and her boy-husband did nothing to improve her situation. He did as his mother wished, and no doubt saw his wife's travails as part of a cultural rite of passage in the centuries-old power play between mother and daughter-in-law. There was no romantic love between my grandparents, at least not the kind of love I would have wanted. Theirs was a love born of familiarity, habit, obligation. My grandfather kept at least one mistress and had at least one child with her, a girl. I'm sure my grandmother knew about them because my grandmother knew everything, but she never spoke of them. When my grandmother died, after nearly sixty years of marriage, my grandfather grieved for her for a brief period of time, and then he went to China to retrieve and marry my grandmother's sister, a widow, who would take care of him in his later years. An excellent example of a man who couldn't cope.

My parents' story was marginally better. My mother was beautiful, truly. In the small town in which I would later be born, my mother's beauty caught my grandmother's eye. Her firstborn son was twenty-four; it was time for him to get married. She asked around about this pretty girl who walked past the house four times a day, back and forth from the school where she taught first grade. Her parents were from Hainan, too, although she had been born in Vietnam. The eldest of six children. Not a rich family but a perfectly respectable family, and her beauty could not be ignored. So my grandmother dispatched a match-maker to my mother's house in Hoi An to broach the possibility of a union. My maternal grandparents were ecstatic. My mother was not. She had seen my father—a pale-skinned man, handsome enough— from a distance. But my mother felt she, at twenty-two, was too young to get married. She longed for adventure. She wanted to work at a different job, something other than teaching, like for the Americans at the army store. But her father wouldn't allow her to mix with the Americans, for doing so was an invitation to corruption, scandal, and ruin.

Her parents pressured her to agree to the marriage. They said that given my father's family's reputation and wealth, my mother might not get a better offer, that marrying well was her single greatest duty to her parents and younger siblings. She agreed, and thus began a brief courtship that had to be organized around the war. My father had been drafted, but my grandmother had bribed enough people to ensure that he would serve as a captain's driver and not fight on the front lines. When he wasn't on duty, he would ride his motorcycle to visit my mother on Saturdays in Hoi An, a two-hour trip that he had to wait to embark on until late morning to ensure that the American and South Vietnamese forces had sufficient time to clear the roads of any land mines that might have been planted overnight by the Vietcong.

My parents married on the sixth day of the eleventh month of the lunar calendar in the Year of the Monkey, also known as Christmas Day 1968. It was chosen because the people who knew such things said it was an auspicious day, a day that portended good fortune and many blessings. They married in Da Nang, with my mother and her family and friends traveling there several days beforehand and staying at a hotel to ensure that the trouble and inconvenience of war—torn-up roads and unexpected skirmishes—would not interrupt the festivities.

When I ask my mother if she loved my father when she married him, she says no; she says that she grew to love him over the years. Theirs was also a love born of familiarity, habit, obligation; a love born of surviving a war, Communism, and emigration together. Growing up, I didn't see the love. Mostly, I saw lots of fighting, primarily my dad yelling at my mom, to the point where I thought he was verbally abusive. Maybe his anger came from the stresses of resettling in a new country, where he was nothing when he had once been something. Things got better through the years, as my father mellowed with age, as my mother grew more confident in this new country and learned to fight back. Nonetheless, I swore that I never wanted that kind of marriage, and certainly not that kind of love.

It didn't seem like my father wanted love for me at all. I once asked him when I was in high school, even as my many Asian friends were sneaking around dating behind their parents' backs, when I could have a boyfriend. He said not until I had graduated college, that all that "boyfriend-girlfriend nonsense" was a distraction from school and that he wouldn't permit such indecency. I remember when we dropped my sister off at Berkeley for her freshman year, as we drove around campus my father would point to the girls wearing skimpy tank tops and makeup, and he'd say with the utmost derision, "Look at those slutty girls." I was just entering eighth grade, but the message was loud and clear. My father wanted me to not be one of those slutty girls. No boyfriends. I had to focus on academic excellence. Since I couldn't drive because of my vision issues, my father always dreamed of becoming my driver one day. He had it all planned out; I could get him a cellphone and buy him a car, and whenever I needed a ride, all I had to do was call him and he would come pick me up and take me wherever I needed to go. My father had endless patience when it came to driving, and driving me in particular. There was never mention of a husband or children in his dream scenario. I vaguely wondered if my father would drive me on dates and evenings out with my friends (for which, horror of horrors, I might dress like a slut).

It wasn't until much later that I realized why there was never mention of a husband or children for me, why my father always stressed education (more with me than with my siblings) and therefore financial independence. It all made sense after my mother told me about my grandmother's failed attempt to have me killed at two months of age, and my parents' complicity in that attempt. Back then, in Vietnam, they were simply trying to save me from a life of miserable blindness, unmarriageability, and childlessness. After all, a girl's worth rested solely on her ability to get married and have children. While it was true that coming to America had saved some of my vision and that in America there was more help and opportunity for people with disabilities, my parents still saw me as a helpless blind baby, deficient, undesirable; to them I was still probably unmarriageable.

I was very broken by the time I left for college at seventeen, and I would continue to be broken for many years thereafter. I was so angry at the universe. Why me? Why did I have to be the one to be blind? Why did I have to be the one to wear ugly, thick glasses? Everywhere I turned, all I could see was what I couldn't do. I couldn't help but also believe that I was defective and deeply flawed. I hated my parents for bringing me into the world and letting me live. I even once hysterically screamed at my father and demanded to know why he had allowed that to happen. Little did I realize how close to home I had hit. Ironically, it was my grandmother who came to calm me. Most of all, I hated myself.

And so even though my romantic self dreamed of you, I never thought I would actually find you or that, if you did exist, you would want me. You've often asked me about the boyfriends I had before you, and I always found ways to evade your questions. The reason is there were no boyfriends before you. Sure, there were dalliances and holiday flings, but the guys never stuck around for more than a few weeks. Maybe they couldn't handle the Williams and Harvard degrees. Maybe my grandmother and parents had been right that no man would want someone as defective as I; it certainly seemed like guys would become exceedingly uncomfortable when they learned of my vision problems. Maybe I believed I wasn't deserving of love, and that my grandmother and parents had been right all along.

I didn't engage in any of the "boyfriend-girlfriend nonsense." No, instead, I put my energies into studying, just like my father wanted me to. But, unwittingly, I also put my energies into fixing what was broken inside me. I packed my bags and left for Williams College, three thousand miles away from home. My dad might have believed that there was no real value in educating a girl and letting me go so far away from home and risking my potential ruin, but he couldn't resist the allure of the college ranked number 1 in the annual *U.S. News & World Report* ratings, and since I had earned a full scholarship, he really had no say in what I did. I studied Chinese, the language my mother thought I could never learn because of my vision. My junior year, I studied in China, traveling around the vast country during every break on as little money as possible. After I graduated college, I studied Spanish in Seville for five weeks and backpacked through Europe alone for another five weeks. The summer after my first year in law school, I did my internship in Bangladesh. After I sat for the bar exam, I traveled to Chile and Peru and then Thailand, and went back to Vietnam for the first time in twenty-three years with my parents. After I started working, I had a few more adventures, to South Africa and New Zealand. And right before I met you, I went to Antarctica, after which I could proudly say that I had been to the seven continents by the time I was thirty.

Somewhere in between having my cabin invaded by squawking chickens on the barge sailing down the Yangzi River, and having the door fly off the bus in some dusty western Chinese province, and praying for my life as we wound down the roads that hug the base of the Himalayas, and camping on the Antarctic ice, and sitting in wonder at the mystic beauty of Machu Picchu, I fixed what was broken inside of me. Nothing could have made me confront my limitations as much as traveling the world did. Nothing could have made me more frustrated or hate myself more than standing on the streets of Rome trying to find a place to sleep for the night while struggling with a map and a magnifying glass. And nothing could have made me more proud of myself and love myself and feel such profound gratitude for what I could do and what vision I did have than kayaking through the Antarctic waters. I learned that no one could tell me what I could or couldn't do, that only I could set my limitations. I learned to appreciate everything that I could do, that indeed even some people with normal vision couldn't have traveled the world alone as I had. I learned to accept myself as I am, to be patient with and love myself.

And then I met you, when I was ready to meet you, when I felt I was deserving of you. Being with you and falling in love with you was the easiest thing I've ever done. It felt so right. You were so smart—my intellectual equal, if not my intellectual superior. You taught me. You challenged me (admittedly sometimes in the most annoying ways). But you know what touched me the most? The way you would wordlessly reach for my hand when we went down a set of stairs, the way you without prompting would start reading a menu to me, the way you happily acted as my driver. You've never doubted my abilities. My sister told me that she warned you right before you were about to Skype with my parents to ask them for permission to marry me (she was going to act as the translator) that you had to accept and love me as I am, visual disability and all. That is exactly what you have always done, loved me and accepted me for who I am with all my imperfections.

It isn't about figuring out how many months after my death would be appropriate. It's about you. My death will break you. It will shatter you into a million little pieces. But I want you and you alone to fix yourself. I want you to use the opportunity to form an incredible bond with the girls that might not have been possible had I lived. I want you to figure out how to manage the kids and the apartment and your career on your own, as lonely as that may feel sometimes. Please don't be with a woman because you need a wife or mother for your children. Know that no woman can make this easier. No woman can fix what is broken inside you. I want you to be whole again through your own doing. And only then do I believe you can find a real, healthy love, someone who is deserving and worthy of you and the girls. Who knows? She might even be someone I would have liked.

I love you, sweetheart. Be well. Until we meet again . . .

Julie

2018

44

The Unwinding of the Miracle

Last year, in May, we were all flying back to New York from Austin. Josh and Mia were in another section and I was entertaining Isabelle, and as we were looking out the window I said, "Belle, wouldn't it be fun if we could just go outside and sit on the clouds?"

And she said "Mommy, don't be silly, you'd just fall right through—it's just air."

And I said, "Do you really think so, Belle? Because, I mean, don't angels sit around on clouds?"

She said, "Do you think angels are real, Mommy?"

"I don't know," I said. "Maybe . . ."

And she said, "Do you think that's what happens after we die, we become angels?" She paused, and thought to herself for a moment, and then quietly said, "I'd like to be an angel."

"Why?" I asked.

"Because otherwise I'd just be dead," she said.

I laughed, and said, "Wow, that's a really good reason."

Wearing a serious expression on her face, my five-year-old then said words that humbled and moved me, words that seem fitting to begin the last chapter of this book. She said, "But for you, mommy, for you, I want you to grow inside another woman's tummy."

Well, as you might imagine, for a time I couldn't speak. Finally, I managed to whisper, "I think that's a wonderful idea, Belle. I hope that happens."

"But Mommy," she said. "Come back well."

My now six- and eight-year-old daughters love having me tell them the stories of how I and they were born. They never tire of hearing the same thing again and again. Of course, the stories couldn't be more different. I used to ask my mother to tell me my story all the time, too.

I was born in the midwife's two-room concrete house, nine months after the fall of Saigon, in a nondescript provincial capital in central Vietnam, which in actuality was nothing more than a little town. The midwife had successfully delivered my father and his four brothers a generation earlier, and had delivered my brother and sister before me (as well as nearly every other baby in the town). There was no prenatal care, no machines, no projected due dates, no epidural. My mother tells me she forgets how bad the pain was. Her stomach hurt the night of the sixth day of the twelfth lunar month of the Year of the Rabbit, and she rode a moped driven by my sister's nanny the few dusty blocks. My father was not home. He was off somewhere trying to sell and deliver the last of our hardware business's inventory before the new regime came to confiscate it and more. My mother lay down, and I came quickly. Nobody recorded the exact time that I entered this world, and my mother doesn't remember.

Both my girls were born at St. Luke's–Roosevelt hospital on Manhattan's Upper West Side. Mia, being the first, required an epidural, twelve hours of labor and an hour and a half of exhausting pushing that so concerned my obstetrician, she finally decided to use a vacuum to remove the baby. With the vacuum, Mia slipped effortlessly out, and within seconds, I was clutching her slippery, wiggling body at 5:56 P.M. Belle came quickly at the height of the summer heat; it was ninety-nine degrees that day, and I was burning up on the street. I was that pregnant lady who couldn't get a cab—shift change or fear of having a pregnant woman deliver in the cab, I couldn't say. So I desperately and impatiently took the subway uptown with my husband, breathing through the excruciating pains as everyone apprehensively looked on, and then walked across two long avenues to Tenth Avenue, where I was greeted by a wheelchair and a security guard who told me to think about ocean waves; I almost told him to shut the fuck up. I was already eight centimeters dilated, so I bypassed the usual admissions process and was rushed into a room where I got an epidural and the doctor broke my water. Belle came resoundingly into the world twenty minutes later at 6:23 P.M.

As ordinary and mundane as new human life is, even my young children, as shown by their insistence on hearing the stories, instinctively recognize that each new human life is anything but ordinary or mundane; they appreciate the uniqueness of each of their birth stories and, by extension, the awesomeness of their existence. Even at their tender ages, they wonder about where they were before they were here and how they came to be. We call it, in all of its triteness, the miracle of life.

A miracle is defined as that which cannot be explained by the laws of science or otherwise defies all known rules of the natural world. The miracle of life in some sense is not a miracle at all. The laws of science can explain how human life comes about—I received those weekly emails from babycenter.com describing what was happening within my womb while I was pregnant—egg meeting sperm, cells rapidly dividing, so many organs forming, so many systems developing. There is no mystery at all. And yet, it is the very creation of life, that undefinable spark that begins the process, that is the miracle. And then from there, a million and one things have to go just right, and fortunately for me and as far as we can tell—knock on wood—they did with respect to my little girls. The proper occurrence of those million and one things in the right time sequence is a miracle. As one who was born blind, I was particularly sensitive to the delicacy of that process that seems so ordinary, how easily something small with far-reaching consequences could go wrong. I suspect I fretted more than the average expectant mother.

These birth stories were what I wanted to write down when I learned that I had Stage IV colon cancer, in 2013; there were so many things, but these most of all. Who else could tell my daughters how I counted their fingers and toes to make sure they were all there? Who else could describe the magic and wonder of seeing them for the first time, their alien-like faces and still-damp, soft skin that strangely smelled of me and them, their nearly bald heads that begged for warmth and nurturing in their utter fragility? The scientific and factual mundaneness of their existence didn't register with me; I could only see them as my little miracles, just as most any mother would. I marveled at the physical aspect of the miracle of life, the feel of skin on skin, the moving limbs, the beating heart of a new life in the world that hadn't been there seconds before.

But there was more that my children needed to understand, which only I could explain to them—the nonphysical aspects, the miraculous parts of their birth stories that involved their very existence, their life stories. Who else could make them understand the truly miraculous nature of their lives and my life, of our lives, inextricably intertwined and shaped by historic and familial forces far beyond our control? Who else could tell them how their births were especially miraculous for me, how insofar as they came from me, their lives could easily have never been, just as mine could easily have never been?

My parents, my grandparents, especially my grandmother, did not see me as a miracle in the physical or nonphysical sense of the word. Quite the contrary. My existence was seen as deeply flawed, a gross failure of whatever miracle of life there was in that forsaken time and place, an abomination, a curse, a problem that had to be addressed in a most drastic manner.

On the bus to Da Nang to have the herbalist give me something that would make me sleep forever, my mother cradled me and quietly wept. She stroked my face. She's so beautiful, she thought. Why must I destroy her? She searched the passing faces, all oblivious to the crime that was about to happen, all smiling and laughing and blithely living life. None of it made any sense to her. Her tears fell like rain onto me.

But between the herbalist, who turned out to be a man of good conscience, and my great-grandmother, who commanded that I be left alone—"How she was born is how she will be!"—my life was saved by a woman I barely remember and a man I never knew. And because my great-grandmother was the ultimate matriarch (the mother of five sons and four daughters, and grandmother and great-grandmother to countless descendants), her decree was the ultimate law in our family. No further attempts were made to end my life. Somehow, despite all, I survived, and I grew.

And then that which seemed impossible in the early days of my life came to pass—I gained vision, imperfect as it is. My mother got me to UCLA, where a young pediatric ophthalmologist, originally from Missouri, who had never seen a case like mine and who warned my mother he didn't know how much vision I would ever have, operated to remove the cataracts. Had I been born in the United States, it would have been an easy matter. But I hadn't been, so it wasn't easy at all. Too many years of cataracts shuttering me from the world had caused my brain to forget the optic nerve pathways that linked brain to eyes, and now my brain didn't know how to use them. Four years old, and my brain was flooded with visual information it could make no sense of. It was too late to teach my brain, even with the best corrective lenses.

But it was more than I had ever had. I could see color and shapes and I could walk on my own and I could read with visual aids and I could watch TV. In time, I would learn to work with the vision I had been given and even thrive despite the severe limitations it imposed. A relatively normal childhood in this new land, family, friendship, academic success, scholarships, elite institutions of higher learning, high-powered career, lots of money, world travels, handsome husband, two beautiful children. All of it came to be despite what my grandmother saw as my future in those early days.

Some might call what happened to me and my life itself a miracle—that is, minus the cancer.

I think a lot about miracles, but not in the context that everyone in the "cancer community" throws about the word, as in hoping for a miraculous cure. I had somehow achieved the impossible in my life. So when I was diagnosed with metastatic colon cancer, many would have argued that if anyone could find a miraculous cure, it would be me. That thought never occurred to me. Rather, when I learned that I had life-threatening cancer, I thought that somehow my grandmother, who had died seventeen years earlier, was trying from the grave to kill me again. I've always felt, even long before I found out about the herbalist, that I have been living on borrowed time, that my life had been saved once already—twice if you count the restoration of residual vision as constructive salvation—that no one gets to have her life saved a third time. Intuitively, I just know that that is how the universe works. No, I haven't been hoping for a miracle. I've already had my miracle and then some. Rather, I've been thinking about the notion of a miracle in the context of life itself—its beginning and ending, my beginning and ending, everyone's beginning and ending, everyone's miracle of life.

When I see myself as having lived on borrowed time all these years, when I take the view that my life was never meant to be, I appreciate anew how my very existence (and therefore my children's existence) is, was, and has always been a miracle. And the cancer, although it is shortening my life, destroying what could have been another forty years of living, in no way diminishes that miracle. Everything that lives must die. Even my small children understand this fundamental rule of nature. Some things just happen to die sooner than expected.

And so, the miracle of life must end for each of us. I happen to know how my miracle will end and am painfully conscious of the fact. And that ending—the how of it, what it will look and feel like, the process of dying, the complete antithesis of birth, the unraveling, the unwinding of the miracle of life, how much of that unwinding is within our orderly control, possessed of a certain beauty, and how much of it is a chaotic undoing of the threads of our lives, ugly and dark—these are the questions that have preoccupied me these past five years, especially now, as the end draws ever closer. But all of it is, in itself, also a miracle.

We live in a culture that fears the unwinding of the miracle. It is dark; it is frightening; it is tragic, especially when the death is deemed premature. When I was diagnosed, I went looking for others like me with whom I could explore the darkness, fear, and tragedy. Processing hard truths and vigorously embracing reality have after all been the salvation of my life. But mostly, I found and continue to find delusion, false optimism, and forced cheer in the face of a devastating diagnosis, where death and all the fears that come with it must be avoided at all cost. Clichés born of that need to avoid the truth—from well-meaning family and friends, but most confoundingly from the sickest and care-givers of the sickest—are unthinkingly offered to me constantly. "There's always hope. You have to stay positive. You have to keep fight-ing. There is no other option." I grit my teeth as I think, Actually, there is a point where there is no more hope for continued life. That's just a factual matter. Really? Why do I have to stay positive? Is there some-thing wrong with being negative? And no, there is always an option, the option of choosing to die. Horror of horrors! In the orthodoxy of dying, this is heresy.

There was the popular blogger who wrote of being excited when she was diagnosed because cancer presented another challenge in her young life and she loved challenges. I felt no excitement when I was diagnosed, and if this woman really had, it was all part of a lie she was telling herself to avoid what was happening in her own body. Another popular blogger only a few short weeks from dying couldn't seem to recognize or accept the telltale signs—the weight loss, the liver invaded by tumors, the five brain metastases. He was a clinician, a cancer re-searcher, which made the denial and delusion that much more as-tounding. The brain tumors were being treated with radiation. Subsequently, as he reported on his blog, he fell over from a loss of balance, which he attributed to inflammation caused by the radiation. He expected the inflammation to subside, and then he would be able to return to systemic treatment. I read and looked at photos he had posted on social media a month earlier, and I knew that there would be no return to systemic treatment. The end was near for him.

Those of us familiar with the cancer world, who have witnessed enough of our friends die, recognized how close he was. He seemed not to be able to see this and perpetuated the delusion to himself as well as to his more naïve blog readers. I was and am disgusted by the lies. Perhaps for many, lying is the only way to get through the day and face death, but I knew that I wasn't one of those people. I wanted to face my death with honesty, with eyes wide open, with understanding and courage even amid the fear, and, I hoped, with some newly gained wisdom. And so I started writing in search of my truth, to gain that understanding and wisdom of what it means to live and die, of what it is to live fully and unwind our individual miracles consciously. I discovered so many others who were secretly looking for their truths, who wanted to explore with me not just the darkness, fear, and tragedy, but also the joy and beauty of living and dying.

The beginning of the miracle of life, the development of the fetus in the womb and then its entry into the world, is associated with wonder and beauty. How unfortunate it is that we all lack the cognition to appreciate that beauty that is the creation of our individual miracle of life. I would have loved to witness my own creation and birth. Now I'm left with witnessing my own death; I have the cognition for that, and as horrible as this disease has become, I hope that I will have the cognition for that, that the complex workings of my brain will be the last functions to shut down. It is hard to find any beauty in dying, any poetic ending to the miracle of my life.

Seven months ago, I failed the second clinical trial in which I had participated and the third experimental treatment overall. It was particularly devastating because the trial had for a couple months showed dramatic efficacy—and then it didn't. The scans revealed doubling and even tripling of certain abdominal and pelvic tumors, a clear portent of obstructions and blockages and eventual death by starvation, unless my lungs or liver failed first from their tumor burdens. I was sure I would be dead within several months. That was the prognosis my oncologist gave me after a five-minute disclaimer. One small part of me was relieved to have the torture end, to finally embark on the next adventure. But mostly I spent the time during what would be my last summer—the summer of 2017—grieving intensely, crying every day for two weeks, realizing again for the umpteenth time with a renewed, intense sadness all the big and small moments I would miss in my daughters' lives—the graduations and weddings and music recitals and fights with friends—as well as all the shattered dreams that my husband and I had once nurtured—a vacation home in Tuscany upon retirement, more travel around the world. You would have thought that I'd never grieved for any of this in the preceding four years.

But there was something new that I did truly mourn for the first time, as I felt my body's unprecedented deterioration as it struggled to continue to operate after four years of surgeries, chemotherapy, radiation, and other experimental treatments, and the undeniable fact of the cancer's progression. Abdominal pain had me permanently hunched over despite the opiates. Bleeding resulting from the cancer's spread to my uterus and vagina was a constant visual and graphic reminder of the cancer. General weakness made me gratefully squat during the short elevator rides to and from my apartment floor when no one else was around. A two-minute trip to the bank became a monumental outing that required mental preparation and then physical and mental stamina. And food—well, that was especially upsetting. I used to love eating, this fundamental affirmative act of life, even through years of chemotherapy. And now I couldn't stand the sight of food, nor could I muster the energy or desire to cook, which I once enjoyed tremendously.

No doubt my body's rejection of this basic need and joy in life was a sign of its desire to not live anymore. I used to be so strong, naturally muscular, and I augmented that natural strength with frequent intense workouts. I used to lug thirty pounds of groceries from Trader Joe's on my back. I used to be able to carry one baby on my back and one in my arms and go up and down stairs. What happened to that woman? She was becoming an ever-distant memory, and I was sad, not for my daughters or my husband, but simply for me, for I realized that I was losing the person who I once was and whom I loved, and this dying woman, this woman who was aging at an accelerated pace, an ugly, ever-thinning creature, was taking her place. As I prepared to die and the invisible wall between me and the living grew thicker and taller, I mourned my own impending death in an ever-shrinking bubble of isolation, loneliness, and darkness.

But then, once my summer of grief was over, my perspective shifted, and a sort of peace came over me. I was sad to be leaving my husband and my daughters, but I felt something else, too: awe at what was happening to my body. I couldn't watch myself be born, but with eyes open, I could watch myself die. And that is no less a miracle than any other. It is hard to find the beauty in dying, but I've learned; I'm learning still.

My grandmother died when I was twenty years old, and it broke my heart because I loved her so very much. My mother told me that my grandmother hated me for a very long time, that she didn't grow to love me until long after we came to this country and I had gained some sight. The odd thing is that when I was growing up, I would have never guessed that my grandmother hated me. She was a wonderful grandmother to all thirteen of her grandchildren, cooking weekly feasts for us and calling us constantly to ask whether we'd eaten dinner yet and coming over to fold our laundry. She had had a hand in raising and caring for each of us at some point in our lives. During the summer before she died (no one, including her, knew she was dying), she and I would take walks in the coolness of the setting sun, her hand grasping my elbow; I was never sure whether she was using me as support or whether she thought she was guiding me; maybe it was a little bit of both. She came with me to the airport to see me off to my senior year of college—she'd never done that before. I remember feeling slightly nervous and nauseous at returning to school after a year of studying abroad and laying my head on her shoulder in the backseat of the car as my dad sped along the freeway at that early hour; I remember hugging her and telling her I'd see her at Christmas and her waving goodbye to me as I boarded the plane.

Seven weeks later I flew home to sit at her hospital bedside as she faced her last days, her skin yellowed, her body bloated, and her ability to speak gone. She was surrounded by her enormous family. Her daughters-in-law would take turns spending the night with her to make sure she was never alone. I was moved by all the love that surrounded her. There was something special about my grandmother, something that drew people to her, even in her darkest days.

I tried unsuccessfully to study for midterms as I tried much harder to process this first death of someone I truly loved, to reconcile this diminished woman who was days from leaving this world with the dominant woman I'd always known, she who had left her little village as a girl to travel by boat to a foreign land where a boy she'd never met waited to marry her, she who had never learned how to read but through her sons and grandchildren found all the success she ever dreamed of, she who had such an iron will that she'd not thrown up once on the fishing boat that took us away from Vietnam even as everyone around her retched into the sea.

At the end of the fourth day of my visit, I went to bid her farewell, knowing that once I left her side that evening I would never see her alive again. The room was filled with her children and grandchildren. I took her hand—it was too warm and as dry as rice paper. Her eyes remained closed, as they were most of the time now. "I have to go back to school tomorrow, Grandma," I said in our Chinese dialect. I wasn't sure she could hear me or if she was even awake. I switched into English then, because I didn't have the words in Chinese, knowing she would understand at least the universal sentiments. "I love you, Grandma. I'm going to miss you so much. And I'm going to make you so proud of me, I promise." In tears, I put her hand back on her stomach and turned away to leave the room, to find a corner in the hallway where I could cry and grieve in solitude. I barely heard the sudden sobs that arose from those in the room as my father grabbed my shoulder and forced me to face my grandmother once more. She'd raised her hand and was waving it ever so slowly back and forth in a gesture of farewell. What that simple act must have cost her in terms of pain endured and energy spent I can only imagine. Understanding that this was her ultimate gesture of love left me crying for days, months, and years afterward.

I've spent the years since my diagnosis grieving and exploring the darkness, but I've also basked in the love and compassion shown to me, not unlike the love shown to my grandmother. I have loved my family and they me much more than if I had not become sick; we've learned to communicate with each other with an intimacy I would have never dreamed possible had life gone the way I had planned. Because of my insistence on honesty in confronting death, my girls show an emotional maturity, compassion, and appreciation for life rarely seen in children of their age. We have traveled far and wide; I oversaw the combination and construction of a beautiful home that my children will grow into for years to come. I've rejoiced in the ordinary, too, the things that others take for granted and even resent—the cooking and the parent-teacher conferences and the forcing of homework and violin practice. I have lived even as I am dying, and therein lies a certain beauty and wonder. As it turned out, I have spent these years unwinding the miracle that has been my life, but on my terms.

Before the light goes out, I would like to say that, Second Wife, I don't hate you. Please love the family that was mine with all your heart. Take care of them, and live out the life for me that I could not.

Mother, Father, I forgive you. And I thank you.

I will see you soon, Grandmother. I have some things to say to you. I have been thinking about them for a long time.

And for any who might be reading this: I am grateful to have had you here, on this journey. I would presume to encourage you to relish your time, to not be disabled by trials or numbed by routine, to say yes as much as you can, and to mock the probabilities. Luxuriate in your sons and daughters, husbands and wives. And live, friends. Just live. Travel. Get some stamps in those passports.

I traveled to Antarctica several years ago. There, in the midst of its vast unearthly beauty, I felt as if I were glimpsing another planet, another dimension, possibly the afterlife. It was a retired widower from Indiana whom I'd met a year earlier during a safari in South Africa who told me he'd been to Antarctica and that it had been a very spiritual experience. That planted the seed in my head, and after a particularly exhausting transaction closed at work in October 2005, I booked a last-minute trip to Antarctica for late November, several weeks ahead of my thirtieth birthday. I went alone (or as alone as you can when going to Antarctica, since there really is no way for the ordinary tourist to get there other than to join a group), making my way down to Tierra del Fuego, the very tip of South America, from which all the Antarctica-bound ships in the Western Hemisphere depart. Together with forty-three other tourists from all over the world, I boarded a Russian ice vessel and embarked on a turbulent two-day crossing of the Drake Passage to reach the Antarctic Peninsula.

On Thanksgiving Day, as we approached land with the ship breaking through sheets of ice that had formed on the water's surface, I stood on deck, gazing in absolute wonder at the massive glaciers in infinite shades of white, blue, and green rising above the water, majestic arches and craggy mountains made of old and new ice sculpted over time, more glorious than anything ever made by any human being. The blue of the cloudless sky, the light of the sun that, at that time of year, shone for twenty hours a day, and the perfect whiteness of the land itself was so intense that it was almost too much to bear.

Over the next seven days, I would escape the noise of the ship to kayak, paddling through the deepest quiet and the silkiest waters, waters that rippled with each stroke, waters that perfectly reflected the sky's mood. Contrary to popular belief, Antarctica is not all white. It is yellow, pink, red, and purple in the light of the quasi rising and setting sun; it is black and gray in the volcanic rock that covers the beaches where the snow has melted for the season. It is orange in the penguin beak, green in the shallow waters, and brown in the seal coat. And to it all, there is a vibrancy, purity, and beauty that never failed to make me breathless and tearful, that made me grateful to whatever gods there may be for having given me sight to behold such magnificence.

In Antarctica, I felt as if we had departed our home planet and were closer to some serious answers about what it all means. One cannot help but think big thoughts in such a place. One cannot help but imagine God—and I use the word *God* to refer not to the one depicted in any religious teachings but rather to a being that may very well be a force comprised of all the life that has been and is and will be, a force that is incomprehensible to the mind but perhaps perceptible to the soul, the way great poetry eludes logic but overwhelms the emotions. And within the shadow of that greatness and grandeur, I felt small, insignificant, a little life spanning a second in time on a little blue planet, in a solar system, in a galaxy, in a universe that goes on forever and ever, an infinitesimal blip in space and time.

Feeling small and insignificant is a rarity in the course of our daily lives. Sure enough, once I returned from Antarctica, I again became consumed by the minutiae of my life, minutiae that often felt important and momentous—navigating family and friend dramas, drafting hundred-page contracts late into the night and vehemently negotiating with opposing counsel over little words as though it all mattered so much, feeling annoyance at the guy who cut me in line, planning a wedding, buying an apartment, agonizing over which crib to buy, battling the kids over teeth brushing and TV watching and on and on with all the stuff of life. We live every day not in the shadow of greatness and grandeur but within the confines of our small but seemingly enormous lives. It is a natural way to be; after all, we must live our lives.

And then things happen that jerk us out of our complacency and make us feel small and powerless again. But I have learned that in that powerlessness comes truth, and in truth comes a life lived consciously.

When the time comes, I will happily and with a great sigh of relief climb into my bed knowing that I will never need to get up again. I will surround myself with family and friends, as my grandmother did. I will eagerly greet the end of this miracle, and the beginning of another.

Epilogue

by Joshua Williams

'd like to begin by saying that I am a much more private person than Julie was. I don't think that it would have ever occurred to me to do what she has done—to leave a chronicle of her life and her illness that lays it all bare, and reveals her story so intimately, to so many. But of course I believed in her so completely, and loved her so dearly, that I became a believer in her writing, my personal feelings aside, no matter how hard it was to sometimes read.

And so now I put the finishing note on this story, just as she asked me to do.

I write this from the room in our apartment, our dream home, where Julie died.

Her hospice bed was right here, here as she said her final goodbyes, here as the cancer finally had its way. It's been three months and four days since that morning—March 19, 2018—a bright late-winter morning. So much living happened in this room before that day, though. Before Julie combined the apartments that became the wonderful home she made for us—she was sick the whole time, it must be said—this room was our master bedroom. Here, in this sun-splashed room, with its view of the Statue of Liberty, Mia and Isabelle were conceived. Here, we looked out at the most dazzling sunsets in New York, and had some of the most intimate conversations of our marriage. Here, feeling flush with the future, we planned our life together.

In the end, here was where we tried our very hardest to make Julie's last days comfortable.

For the entire last year, Julie had been leaving us in stages. The mets were increasing, everywhere. By late fall, she had had several bouts of pneumonia, and we discovered that she had a new tumor in her lung the size of a peach, which she chose to have irradiated, just to buy some more time. Even so, we knew that Thanksgiving would be the last Thanksgiving. Christmas would be the last Christmas. Her birthday in early January 2018 would be her last birthday. The pace of her decline was accelerating, and in the end stage of metastatic disease, the stage known as active death, the life leaves you by the hour, and the pain increases exponentially. To keep up, the home hospice aides had to increase her pain medications to astonishing doses just to keep her as comfortable as possible.

Monday, February 26—exactly three weeks before Julie died—is a day that will always haunt me. As she became ever sicker, Julie was prescribed a dizzying array of pain medications, and during the weekend before that day it was clear to me for the first time that Julie had become somewhat incoherent. Seeing this shook me deeply, not just because I finally understood the horrifying truth that her life was almost over, but because no matter how much her body had betrayed her or how brutal a particular treatment might have been, the power of her mind had until then been entirely undiminished. Seeing Julie struggle to figure out what day it was, watching her fumble with names, hearing her speak in a whispery voice that was so profoundly unlike hers—those things were, in themselves, utterly devastating. I tried to squelch the panic rising in me, and by searching her phone I was able to figure out that Julie had an appointment scheduled with her palliative care team at Memorial Sloan Kettering for that very afternoon.

By the time we got to the hospital, Julie had rallied and was her normal self, and we sat together in the small room at MSK and waited to see Dr. R.S., the head of her pain management team. As a palliative oncologist, Dr. R.S. encounters an emergency in every room he enters.

And yet he is a man who radiates goodness without fail. Taking me aside in the hall, he gently told me that it was "a matter of weeks, not months." It turned out that he had just said the same thing to Julie, and when I walked back into the room where she was still quietly perched on the examination table, she and I locked eyes in a way that I will never forget. With that single look and without a word, we both knew that it was over.

Dr. R.S. and his team sent Julie directly to the hospital for what was to be the final time. I remember how she wept in the examination room, how she said she wanted to go home to be with the girls, Chipper, and me. Julie didn't cry easily, God knows, and so I saw it as my main objective at that point just to get her home, no matter what it took. She had planned this part of her illness meticulously, and her plan did not include being hooked up to machines in a hospital. She wanted to die here, at home, in this room.

But first, her oncologist and palliative care team had to get her pain under control and assess her quickly changing condition, to determine how best to make sure that her last days were tolerable without the intravenous medications that only a hospital setting could afford her. With no time to waste, the doctor told us, very bluntly: Get the home hospice team in place, quickly. Make final preparations, now. It was time.

The morning after her hospitalization, Julie was foggy from the opioids, which meant that she was functioning merely at a normal adult level of cognition. And she was tearful, we both were, as it became clear to us that the end that we had been contemplating and fighting against and surrendering to for close to five agonizing years was now upon us. "How can I die?" she asked searchingly. "How can I be dying?" She repeated the questions over and over that morning, between sobs. The words in those questions took on every conceivable meaning—they were both procedural and philosophical. *How can this be happening to me?* she seemed to be asking. And, how does one go about dying, in the practical sense? *How do I do this?* They were, of course, thoroughly logical and reasonable questions, very Julie questions to ask, and at that moment the only questions left to consider. Because, of course, Julie had already seen to everything else.

She had taken care of every last detail for me and the girls, every-thing except: How were we supposed to go on living without her?

Well, from where I sit in this place where she lived so vividly, I can say that there is no good answer to that question. And I suspect that there never will be.

One of the things I most want you to know is that Julie died just as she wanted to die. She was surrounded by the people she loved most in the world—her parents; her sister, Lyna; brother, Mau; beloved cousins Nancy and Caroline; my parents and sisters. And, of course, Mia, Isabelle, and me. One week before the end, on the evening of March 12, we invited people from every stage of her life to our home and held a vigil, just as she'd asked. She lay on the couch in the living room as Mother Kate from our church led the room in prayers and moments of meditation, and one by one, the people who had gathered around her told stories of Julie's life—of her life as a college student, or as an intrepid world traveler, or as a class mom, or as a fellow cancer patient, or as a writer—and we laughed and we cried and we ate and we drank. All except Julie, that is. She had stopped eating, and would never eat again.

During the vigil, the hospice team showed up with her bed, and they discreetly set it up in the room where I now sit. That was the first night Julie would spend in that bed, which marked the night before as the last night we would sleep in the same bed.

To say that I was terrified at what was to come does not convey the depth of my terror, but to say that I also wished fervently for an end to Julie's suffering—in spite of myself—well, my words are truly inade-quate to describe the size of that moment. But those opposite emo-tions that I felt give you an idea of the confusion that the imminent death of the most important person in your life brings on. When you are as sick as Julie was, deliverance becomes an act of mercy.

Nothing can prepare you for what happens after death.

Numbness initially protects you from the crushing power of for-ever, and so in the first weeks and even months after Julie left us, there was a jarring lightness to life. All the shoes had dropped, the ceaseless nightmare of terminal disease was over, and the horror of watching the person you most love in all the world suffer terribly abruptly stopped. Five years of frenzy and fear, suddenly gone. To say that it was unexpected and counterintuitive to feel happiness and even moments of real joy as notions of the future for me and Mia and Belle began to creep into my consciousness would be beyond understatement. I was shocked by these feelings, and found myself taking long walks in Fort Greene Park as spring came on, allowing myself to begin to process all of it, really for the first time. Living with the constant emergency of terminal illness doesn't give you the chance to do that. Instead, you function moment to moment, day to day, maybe week to week. Beyond that, there is no future. And then, suddenly, there was a future, slowly spreading out before us.

At first, this was surprising, and quite a relief. "This isn't so horrible," I thought to myself on more than one occasion. And then, just as suddenly, the anesthetic effect of trauma begins to wear off, and the deep pain of permanent loss begins to set in. That point, a couple of months after Julie died, I now recognize as when real grief well and truly began. For a time, I was incapacitated with grief, and a flood of unprocessed emotions, haunted by regret, self-doubt, and an unhealthy dose of demon guilt.

One of the real blessings of my life is that almost every Sunday, I talk to my father for an hour on the phone. I feel very lucky to have his wise counsel. As the full weight of what had happened hit me, I called my dad.

I was being torn apart by the guilt and feelings that I had not done enough for Julie, consumed by a flood of thoughts, not all of them very rational. I found myself relentlessly going back to 2013 in my mind, and looking at pictures of Julie from the spring of that year, just before her diagnosis, marveling at her beauty and youth and vitality, and her unfettered joy and limitless possibility, even as I now knew that inside of her a killer was loose.

I told my dad, "Look I'm really hurting. I think I fucked it up. I think I didn't do enough to save my wife. I should have been able to see this back in 2010 or 2011, or certainly in 2012. But I didn't. I failed Julie."

And my father said, essentially, You think you have that kind of power, do you? The truth is, there was nothing you could have done. You might not ever be able to reconcile that Julie was at the same time young and vital and also doomed—that it was too late, from the start. But for your own sake and the sake of the girls—for Julie's sake— you've got to try.

The die had been cast. Julie's death had been inexorable. Control, an illusion. All else—all the scrambling, the working of the odds, the second, third, and fourth opinions, the clinical trials, the alternative therapies, and on and on—all were just the rituals strewn along the path to the inevitable.

But that—*cancer kills*—is hardly a revelation. The revelation would come in how Julie responded to her fate. For the little girl born blind, she saw more clearly than any of us. In facing the hard truth of her terminal illness, and never averting her gaze or seeking refuge in fantasy, she turned her life into a lesson for us all in how to live fully, vividly, honestly.

For all my fidelity to the numbers that ended up being so brutally accurate—sitting in Julie's darkened recovery room after her first surgery in the summer of 2013, poring over the available studies on Stage IV survival rates by the glow of my iPad—I still did not want to believe or concede to those numbers. And for all her belief in the power of the intangibles that had made her whole life possible, Julie's fidelity was always to the truth, whatever that might be and wherever that might lead. She might have believed a bit in magic, but she never indulged in magical thinking.

And so my father's advice was a welcome salve at a very hard moment. There was, in the end, nothing that could have been done. Moreover, in the end, the recognition of the inevitable had been an article of faith for Julie, too, and apart from leaving Mia and Isabelle, she harbored absolutely no regrets. In the course of this experience, we resolved together to deal in reality—especially in the face of the cottage industry of denial that exists among some in the "cancer community"—but Julie was the exemplar of reality. In our life together I learned so many lessons from her, but none more so than this: It is in the acceptance of truth that real wisdom and peace come. It is in the acceptance of truth that real living begins. Conversely, avoidance of truth is the denial of life.

Julie had faced more hard truths than anyone I will ever know. More hard truths than in any three lifetimes. So she was very wise indeed, well before her grandmother's colon cancer came stalking her at the age of thirty-seven. And through her writing, she came to process her own life of struggle and in so doing became empathy itself, providing a vocabulary to an ever-widening community of people living their lives and struggling to face their own hard truths.

Once, in thinking about what it was she most wanted this book to be, she wrote:

> To the degree that my book speaks truth about not just the cancer experience but the human experience in general, I want people to be able to find themselves in the writing. And in so doing, I want them to realize that they have never been and will never be alone in their suffering. . . . I want them to find within the rich, twisted, and convoluted details of my life truth and wisdom that will bolster and comfort them through their joys and sorrow, laughter and tears.

And so now I face my own hard truth. That is to a great degree where committing Julie's legacy to the page, and creating a record of her extraordinary life, comes in. Turning my attention to memorializing her story so that it will live on feels very purposeful, and is a way to engage the grief, conjure the memories, and come to terms with the fact that although she is gone, she will always live on, here, in the eternal present, taking me and her daughters, and you, too, by the hand, and telling you the most remarkable story. This becomes all the more important as the days and years and decades inevitably accumulate, life sweeps us all further down the river, and memory erodes. When I think about that happening, I am even more grateful for Julie's writing.

In the spirit of that writing, and so that others who are going through ordeals similar to ours might not feel so alone in their suffering, before I finish here I feel that I must mention the toll that disease takes on even the best relationships. As deeply connected and profoundly committed as Julie and I were for the entirety of our time together, as death approached our paths diverged sharply. As she contemplated death and what comes next, I contemplated our daughters and the devastating prospect of life without and beyond Julie. The growing distance had the effect of making us seem alien to each other, like strangers flailing in the face of eternity. We became the focus of each other's despair. It was often unbearable, and like many couples similarly trapped, we fought terribly and repeatedly. It got so bad that each of us threatened to leave at various times. Divorce was mentioned, brutal things were said. Such is the hurricane of terminal disease—it destroys not only the afflicted, but everyone and everything in its path as well.

But we didn't leave. We didn't divorce. Pulling back from such a brink when it feels that all in your life is spinning out of control requires an effort that can seem beyond you. But that is what Julie and I did. We faced that hard truth together, reaffirmed the reasons that had brought us together in the first place, and said all the things to each other that needed to be said.

The last months of her life and of our life together were lived in tender, loving appreciation. We held hands, we watched our favorite television shows, we fell asleep on the couch together. We did the thing that I most enjoyed in this world, which was simply spending time with her, however I could.

As I mentioned at the outset, I am Julie's opposite in that I am not a public person. My reticence in that regard extends to Mia and Isabelle, too. They are such lovely young women, curious and kind, each possessed of Julie's intellect and empathy. I will always try my best to live up to Julie's standards for them, and to impart Julie's love to them. They are coping with her absence in understandable and different ways. And on May 5, at our church in Brooklyn, each bravely got up before a roomful of people who had assembled for Julie's memorial service and performed music for their mother—Mia on violin and Belle on piano.

And somewhere, Julie was listening, her eyes closed tightly, all the better to hear.

I love you to eternity, sweetheart. Until I see you again.

June 2018

Acknowledgments

We will forever be grateful to many people, both for taking such loving care of Julie's story and for taking such loving care of Julie and our family during the most trying times imaginable.

Thank you to Mark Warren of Random House, who was Julie's editor but more important was Julie's friend. Mark saw the distinctive power in Julie's writing, and their long conversations gave this book its final shape. Thanks also to Julie's fierce advocate, her literary agent, David Granger, who believed in this book before we knew a book was possible, and had the grace to remove his shoes as he entered our apartment (Julie couldn't get over that). And, very importantly, sincere thanks to everyone at Random House, Julie's literary home—in particular Andy Ward and the extraordinary marketing and publicity team, to whom Julie was very close—Leigh Marchant, Maria Braeckel, Michelle Jasmine, and Andrea DeWerd—and to production editor Evan Camfield, who took such wonderful care with Julie's writing.

There are too many individuals to name, and so we do hope that the extraordinarily talented and dedicated medical professionals who treated and cared for Julie—from her first surgery at UCLA to NYU and Memorial Sloan Kettering—know just how grateful we are and will always be to them. We simply could not have asked for kinder or more patient or more intelligent attention, not just to Julie but to our whole family.

We would like to thank Mother Kate and the entire community at St. Ann & the Holy Trinity Church for taking us in when we most needed it.

Julie felt and Josh feels such deep gratitude for the law firm where Julie worked—Cleary Gottlieb Steen & Hamilton—and to Josh's firm as well—Akin Gump Strauss Hauer & Feld. After Julie's diagnosis in 2013, she didn't work another day, but still Cleary kept her office for her, and her assistant remained dedicated to her for the rest of her life. Additionally, early on, Cleary held a fundraiser in Julie's name, the proceeds of which went to colorectal cancer research. Julie's diagnosis came just as Josh had made partner, which in and of itself can be a pretty stressful time. But Akin Gump made it clear to our family that what mattered most was Julie's health, Mia and Isabelle's well-being, and our collective peace of mind. We cannot say enough to thank these two firms for their kindness and support.

We cannot adequately express our thanks to the small town that lives in our Brooklyn apartment building—from perfectly timed covered dishes that kept us fed to perfectly timed offers of babysitting to just the wonderful companionship of the best neighbors a family could ask for, we are beyond grateful. Mia, Isabelle, and Josh will do their best to reciprocate the neighborliness.

We would like to thank Josh's mom and Julie's mother-in-law, Beck Williams, for her selfless and tireless service to Julie and the girls during the hardest moments. She would leave home for weeks at a stretch to come stay in Brooklyn to take Julie to chemotherapy, or just to keep her company. For that, we will be forever grateful.

We would be remiss if we did not thank perhaps the most important people to this enterprise: Julie's readers. This book represents a dream come true for Julie, and the dream would have been impossible without you. Whether you read Julie's blog or heard of her story elsewhere and have come to her writing here for the first time: Thank you for being here. You have our deepest gratitude. May her memory live on through all of us.

Last but not least, we also want to thank Michael Sapienza and everyone at the Colorectal Cancer Alliance (ccalliance.org). Julie believed in this group, supported its work, and subscribed to its mission, which is nothing short of a cure.

About the Author

Born in Vietnam, JULIE YIP-WILLIAMS was a writer, mother, wife and lawyer who grew up in California and graduated from Harvard Law School. In July 2013 she was diagnosed with stage four colon cancer. She died in March 2018, aged forty-two, and leaves behind her husband, Josh, and their daughters, Mia and Isabelle.